Banish Belly and Lose Weight In Just Five Minutes a day!

A Simple Solution To America's Weight Problem

No diet, drug or vigorous exercise to risk your health

Dr. Sukhraj S. Dhillon, Ph. D.

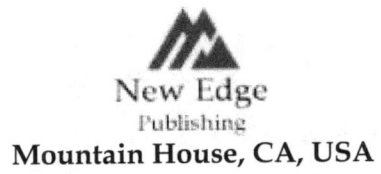

New Edge
Publishing
Mountain House, CA, USA

Other Titles and their ISBNs under Self-help and Spiritual Series:
"The Power of Breathing" (ISBN: 978-1466371545)
"A Simple Solution to America's Weight Problem" (ISBN: 978-1466377127)
"Art of Stress-Free Living:" (ISBN: 1413795064)
"Forever Young" (ISBN: 978-1466392069)
"A New Look at Vegetarianism:" (ISBN: 1575150298)
"Health, Happiness & Longevity:" (ISBN: 0870405276)
"Soul and Reincarnation" (ISBN: 978-1466395930)
"Science, Religion & Spirituality" (ISBN: 1424111269)
"In Search of God" (ISBN: 978-1466398498)
"A Treasure of Great Spiritual Stories" (ISBN: 978-1466394773)
"Industrial Leaks and Air Pollution:" (ISBN: 9997691547)
"Cigarette Smoking:" (ISBN: 9997691547)

First Printing: September 2011

ISBN-13: 978-1466377127
ISBN-10: 1466377127

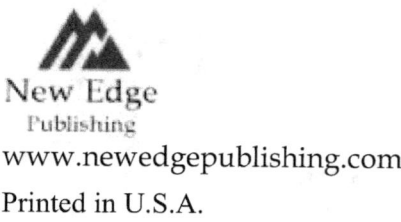

New Edge
Publishing
www.newedgepublishing.com
Printed in U.S.A.

Contents

Introduction

More than half of all American adults are overweight and it's hard to turn on the TV without encountering a commercial for another weight loss remedy. This growing epidemic of obesity has not spared even the young school children who are showing high blood pressure, and other psychological and social problems related to overweight. The latest data shows one-third youngsters and two-third adults are obese (Time, September 12, 2011).

Many of us know that to maintain a desirable weight is good, not only in terms of good looks, but more importantly, in terms of good health. However, the relationship between proper weight and health is more complicated than you think. The scales and scientific methods for calculating overweight and over all fat amounts are important, but more important in terms of health is where you carry the fat more than how much extra fat you carry. Add to this a new study in 2009 which shows that brown fat, same as baby fat, in fact can help lower weight; it's white fat that is the culprit. One of our aims is to tackle the fat problem, and to provide an effective technique to lose weight. Overweight or obesity is probably one of the most important dietary problems talked about and written about today. Over 30 billion dollars are spent annually on weight reduction efforts in the United States, and the 30 billion dollar figure does not include the medical costs resulting from obesity-related diseases.

All kind of diets, exercise programs and other solutions have not worked even though it has become a billion dollar industry. If it did, we will not have all these grim statistics and over-weight people walking around. You will read some of the real stories by real people struggling to maintain proper weight.

This book goes beyond the traditional solutions and describes the very personal secret that I am sharing for the first time. The secret that is most effective among any method I have tested or written about weight loss.

I have known whatever is to know about weight, health, yoga, meditation from East as well as from West. Because I have an advanced degree in science in the west at Yale University in USA and had my earlier education in the East at Punjab University in India. I have written 12 guides combining Eastern and Western approach to total health from stress-free living and spirituality to vegetarianism, happiness and longevity.

However, I could not reduce even 5 pounds with typical diet and exercise. Look below my daily eating habits and other life style that many of us including medical and scientific experts can call ideal. Here it is my typical day:

After getting up in the morning: 1 cup of tea with no sugar but little skim milk

Breakfast: ¼ cup Oatmeal cereal

Snack: Apple, Banana or other fruit

Lunch: About one cup Frozen Vegetables microwaved, plus egg-white from boiled egg.

Evening Snack: Mostly Tea only [rarely a bran muffin].

Supper: Two whole wheat (or millet) chapattis equivalent to about 2 slices of bread. Vegetable cooked Indian style with spices and little oil.

Drink plenty of water, 2 cups skim milk/soymilk, no soda, no alcoholic drink (except in a company or at a party).

Exercise: About 5-10 minutes of yoga stretches in the morning. 3-4 miles walk in the evening.

This schedule is quite healthy and have kept me disease free, pain free, and youthful in all aspects so far in my 60s now.

You will wonder what is left to tell that can reduce weight and stomach after following the above schedule. I was thinking the same till I tried something very simple and very effective. That's what I will share for the first time in this book. It can be done anywhere, anytime and requires no special equipment. And this is not even any diet or vigorous exercise or some nutrient, vitamin, hormone, and drug that I am promoting.

The book is divided in three parts. Part one is about diet concept using the best of eastern traditions and western scientific knowledge. However, the traditional dieting approaches, in general, have not worked, and the number of over-weight young and old have gone up. We suggest you read this useful information. But may quickly go through this part if not have time or not interested in dietary aspect. Part two is actual technique that needs to be understood as thoroughly as possible. Part three describes the science behind the technique and technicalities. The reader is suggested to read part three primarily to understand the theory and to master the technique. If not interested in theory or don't have time, you may again quickly go through part three. But we highly recommend you read it.

Finally remember "your body is a temple of the soul and the holy spirit, a gift from God." Consider every day what you can do to Care for the Temple. With child obesity rates at national health emergency levels (that has involved first lady Michelle Obama now), it is time to treat those fat, unhealthy, undisciplined, drug infested bodies like a temple. This book is here to help you with that. Good Luck!

PART I

1

Diet Concept and Other Traditional Approaches; Why Do These Fail

This part describes the traditional approaches such as diets and exercise programs. We have focused only on the latest and most effective of such programs. But in general these programs require lot more discipline and frustrate most of the overweight people. That is why liposuction and stomach-stapling has become popular quick fix.

More Fruits and Veggies

Weight problems are rare in populations where a lot of natural fruits, vegetables and whole grains are consumed. But excess weight is a common problem in developed countries like the United States, where the progress of scientific and technical development has led to the common use of processed and refined foods, as well as use of growth hormones for profitable animal farming. One of the obvious effects of this move is the high caloric intake resulting from the decreased volume of processed foods. In other words, over-consumption of calories to fill the stomach, which leads to an overweight. Traces of growth hormones from farm animals is also a contributing factor for the overweight problem.

More fruits and vegetables makes sense and that's why one of the dietary aspect of overweight include the effectiveness of fruits, vegetables and whole grains to handle this twentieth century problem. Totally vegetarian diets are best at successfully modifying eating habits in a way that produces lasting results. People who lost weight have admitted that fruits and vegetables was their biggest secret of weight loss and weight maintenance. However, many doctors make a mistake to recommend moderate diets because they believe patients will cheat on strict diets or give up on them entirely. But research shows dieters are more likely to follow strict diets than moderate ones. The reason is that the diet regime is clear-cut, so cheating can't be rationalized. And ... strict diets bring faster results-and with them the vital positive reinforcement of visible success. Moreover, fruits and vegetables are staple foods in many cultures and can provide a tasty alternative. These should not be treated as diets.

We do not suggest that you become a vegetarian and give up meat completely. However, you will find out that how much advantage vegetarian-foods provide in terms of calories. So that concentrating on wholesome vegetarian-foods can make it much easier to diet. The effectiveness of a wholesome vegetarian diet in weight control could be due to several reasons. First of all, wholesome diets with lots of fruits and vegetables are simply low in calories and saturated fat but high in health promoting minerals and vitamins. Secondly, the fiber content in wholesome vegetarian foods gives the dieter a feeling of fullness in the stomach, which reduces the appetite. Studies on a high fiber diet also claim that it requires more chewing. Chewing (mastication) diminishes the sensation of abnormal appetite that compels a person to eat more than is needed. This results in a diet that responds only to natural hunger. It is possible that because of the decrease in bowel transit time caused by the high fiber content of natural foods, small amounts of the fat and protein you eat are excreted. Therefore, a few of the calories you eat really don't count. High fiber content may also inhibit absorption of nutrients through the intestine, thus encouraging weight loss. Although some of the nutrients not absorbed may be categorized as "essential," the consumption of protein and other nutrients by most Americans is so much in excess of what is needed that this degree of loss is not likely to be a problem.

An additional advantage of vegetarian foods is that you don't consume animal growth hormones that come from meat consumption. One of the reasons for American weight problem is the growth hormones in meat and poultry. That is the hormones that are used on animal farms for faster growth of the stock. If you're not strict vegetarian then to lose weight, eat meat and poultry that is grass fed, ideally kosher, and most importantly, has not been given growth hormones. The fish you eat should not be farm raised.

Considering the overweight problem and weight-consciousness of Americans, however, it is surprising that more people have not moved towards vegetarians foods- perhaps lack of awareness about vegetarian nutrition and cooking has been a major contributing factor. As you may know, vegetables are very low in calories and high in health-promoting natural minerals and vitamins; and their bulk fills the stomach and thus satisfies the appetite. For example, 5 ounces of meat provides 500 calories, whereas the same amount of cooked kidney beans provides only 167 calories. Green beans and other fresh vegetables are even lower in calories, and on the average provide less than one fourth of the calories than that of kidney beans. A lunch of vegetable soup, a slice of wholegrain bread, cottage cheese and fruit salad has a third fewer calories than a typical cheeseburger lunch (and far, far less saturated fat and cholesterol). And for the caloric value of a 6-ounce steak, a vegetarian could eat 3 cups of rice or a whole pound of noodles or, to be more reasonable, the vegetarian could eat a very generous serving of a casserole of noodles, vegetables, and cheese, which would eliminate the need for the potatoes and carrots in the steak dinner. A meal of a cup of brown rice and lentils, two slices of whole-grain bread (or a large baked potato) with buttery spread such as benecol, 1/2 cup each of carrots and peas, a lettuce and tomato salad with dressing, and fruit salad containing a banana, one apple, one orange, 2 tablespoons of raisins, and half a dozen walnuts, would contain about 890 calories (610 less than the steak dinner) and leave the diner positively stuffed. While this is not typical of a meal that might be prepared by an experienced vegetarian, it does illustrate the huge amounts of food a vegetarian can consume without exceeding the body's caloric needs.

In fact following the diet tips presented here, it is not necessary to become a health nut and weigh, measure, and analyze every mouthful of food. It is simply true that you are unlikely to grow fat by including good amounts of fresh vegetables and fruits in your diet. Most of these are over 80 percent water and contain only the smallest traces of fat and very little carbohydrate. A young group of vegetarians studied in Boston weighed on average 33 pounds less than the meat-eating comparison group, because as mentioned earlier, a vegetarian diet is bulky and filling, and it's hard to eat more calories than your body burns. As a result, most people lose weight when they start a vegetarian diet. Those who are strict vegetarians (vegans) and eat no dairy products or eggs may actually have a hard time consuming enough calories to maintain their weight. Clearly, for an obese person a vegetarian diet with its naturally lower caloric content is a blessing. However, a normal (or underweight) person does need to make some adjustments in both total food intake and intake of adequate amounts of foods such as legumes, cereals and nuts to add calories for achieving an appropriate caloric balance. Fish and poultry or small amounts of lean meat are appropriate additions for non-vegetarians.

To suit the wide range of tastes and dietary habits of Westerners, meat analogues may be included to replace meat. Meat analogues are made with soybeans, molded into common meat foods such as sausages and burgers. You may find some of the analogues to be attractive, economical, and healthy alternatives to meat.

Even if you have no interest in vegetarianism, there's no reason why you should have animal protein at every meal or even every day. By including vegetarian dishes in your daily menu and adapting the vegetarian approach to menu planning, you can greatly reduce your dependence on animal protein and especially on high-fat, high-calorie meats.

CAUTION: If you have eaten vegetarian foods in Indian restaurant or Indian house hold, you may be surprised. How unhealthy some vegetarian meal can be! Most of the Indian and even Chinese cooking involve deep frying or some kind of frying in fat—oil or butter. Vegetarian *pakora* and *samosas* are perhaps one the worst foods. These are deep fried and often wrapped in refined flour. All carbohydrates and lot of fat, but hardly any protein.

Even for typical vegetarian dishes, cheese and high calorie salad dressings can add hidden calories and should be used very cautiously.

Diet Plan that can Make you Slim, Not Hungry

As you know from the preceding pages, the natural diet containing wholesome foods of plant origin is generally low in fat, cholesterol and caloric values, but high in stomach-filling bulk such as fiber, and in health promoting natural vitamins and minerals. The following pages will include diet plans mainly as guidelines. Although these are confined for the most part to natural vegetarian foods, fat free lean meats (fish, poultry, lean beef) and meat analogues may be included in small amounts as a supplement.

To follow the diet plan you can easily improvise your own menu for the day from the listed food groups (for 1000 calorie diet of various food groups). As a rule of thumb, include foods from the first three groups varying from 1 to 4 servings depending on individual weight status. This is an example of how to select various food groups to choose a diet of 1,000 calories which provides 53 grams of protein. For maximum weight loss with an intake of 600-700 calories, choose one serving from group 1 and two from each of groups 2 and 3. From the vegetable and fruit groups 4 and 5 choose about 4 servings. In fact, the foods from groups 4, 5 and 6 are so low in calories that they can be eaten in relatively unlimited amounts. To keep from being hungry these unrestricted foods help the dieter avoid the temptation to deviate by providing a satisfying sense of bulk while adding very few calories.

Here's an example for selecting a 1000 calorie diet from various food groups.

Food Group	Approx. Serving Size	Number of Servings	Calories	Protein (grams)	Carbs (grams)	Fat (grams)
1 **Dairy** (fat free) **Products**	1 Cup	2	160	16	24	-
2 **Grains & Starchy Vegetables**	1 slice or 1/2 cup	4	280	8	60	-
3 **Legumes***	1/2 cup	3	300	21	60	5
4 **Vegetables**	1/2 cup	No Limit (4)	100	8	20	-
5 **Fruits**	Equivalent of 1 apple	No Limit (4)	160	-	40	-
6 **Beverages and Seasonings**	As desired	No Limit	0	-	-	-
		Total	1,000	53	204	5

*One 4 oz. serving of fish or fowl without skin may replace one of the legume servings.

Unless there is a serious weight problem, weighing of food is not necessary as long as you are eating plenty of natural foods, particularly from groups 4 and 5 with the added taste of seasonings from group 6. As you may notice, the fat food group is not added. In addition to the natural fat provided by the foods themselves, most of the cooking requires frying in vegetable oils such as corn, cottonseed, safflower, soy, sunflower, and olive oil which will provide enough fat.

A variety of vegetables (for vegetarian recipes see Dhillon, Health Happiness and Longevity: Eastern and Western approach. Japan Publications, Tokyo/Harper & Row, New York, 1983/ **Also available in eBook edition 2009**) can lead you to new, interesting, low-calorie dishes of excellent taste which can keep you slim and healthy for the rest of your life. However, cooking vegetables requires a great deal of time in preparation for peeling, slicing, chopping, etc. You can cut down the time by cooking extra quantities and storing in your freezer. Unlike many diet books, sample menus are not provided here. Taste is a personal choice and, perhaps like you, I do not like someone to tell me what to eat. As long as you follow the guidelines to include foods from all the six groups mentioned in the example above with special emphasis on groups 4 and 5, you do not have to count calories or follow any sample menus. Compulsively counting calories and rigidly following sample menus of foods you do not like is not a part of the diet philosophy that you want to follow for maintaining proper health.

Few Basic Rules for Healthy Eating Habit

Always remember that we 'eat to live' and do not 'live to eat'.

Try to understand the nutritional values of food and-without becoming a diet freak-keep in mind the effects of various foods on your health.

Proper eating should be established, and regularly observed. However, do not eat just because it is meal-time unless you feel you need food.

Do not eat immediately before or after exercise or immediately after physical work or a hurried walk.

Do not involve yourself in hard mental work for at least 15 minutes before and after meals. If tired, relax for 10-15 minutes before eating. Pleasant conversation or relaxed mood while eating is good; arguing or concentrating on the day's problems is harmful.

Drinking pure water with food helps digestion. However, cut down at meal-times; drink about half an hour before or after a meal. Fruit juices are good, but fresh tea will cause no harm.

Cleaning the mouth before and after meals is a healthful habit and keeps teeth healthy.

The teeth are the proper organs of mastication, and every particle of food that requires mastication should be subjected to this operation. Proper mastication saves the stomach from an extra burden.

Slow eating is a good habit and food should be taken into the system no faster than it can be thoroughly chewed.

Mastication and slow eating are considered desirable in promoting health because they help in digestion and also in weight loss by diminishing any sensation of abnormal appetite. Fruit, whole grains, and raw vegetables-essentials of a good vegetarian diet-take a lot more chewing than meat and white bread. Besides being important for healthy teeth, thorough chewing stimulates secretion of saliva and gastric juices, which aid digestion. Poor digestion results in a disordered stomach.

Emphasis on digestion of food seems curious to most Westerners because their common high meat diets with low fiber content are easy to digest. However, in view of the fiber fad, digestion and upset stomach due to high fiber consumption can be a problem. Therefore, gradual increase of fiber intake only from natural foods (and not the added fiber) and proper mastication of these foods are strongly suggested. If you happen to use a mild alcoholic beverage at meal times, it can help in digesting high-fiber foods. However, remember that excessive consumption of alcohol not only adds calories, but can also be addictive.

Cooking Methods

Some cooking methods such as deep frying can add extra calories and fat content to your diet. For example, a 3.5 oz (100 gram) baked potato provides 85 calories and 1% fat, whereas the same amount of French fries provides 214 calories and 42% fat.

There are some substitutes for frying in butter or oil that is worth considering. For frying on the stove top, use a nonstick skillet without fat to fry patties, potatoes, pancakes, French toast etc. For oven frying use a nonstick baking sheet without fat to oven fry breaded chicken, eggplant, patties etc. Replace oil or fat with compatible liquids like cooking wines. Even when cooking is done using fatty foods or fat is added for cooking, you can reduce fat intake: Chill the foods (such as soup and stews) and remove the fat from the top of the container. You can pour stock through several thicknesses of cheese-cloth to remove any remaining fat. If there is no time to chill, you can remove fat by dropping ice cubes in the cooked food and remove the cubes with fat sticking to them. These are just some of the simple suggestions that can lower your intake of fat and calories. You can modify these suggestions and develop new methods that are appropriate for your particular situation.

We may point out that barbecuing, grilling, or smoking-can produce possible cancer-causing substances. One way to protect against them is to wrap food in foil before barbecuing or to put it in a pan to reduce its direct contact with the smoke and flames. You can also raise your grill further above the coals or flame and cook foods more slowly at a lower temperature.

In conclusion, you should choose one of the following methods of cooking -- baking, roasting, oven-broiling, microwave cooking, boiling, steaming, poaching, or stewing. The methods you should not use too often are -- barbecuing, charcoal-broiling, grilling, smoking meats, or frying at high temperatures. Deep frying in saturated fat is big no no.

Do's and Don'ts of Foods and Diet Plans

Proper nutrition is one of the most effective means to reduce the risks of serious health problems. For example, proper nutrition can reduce the risk of heart-related diseases either directly by reducing cholesterol intake or indirectly by controlling weight through proper eating habits.

Here are some important dietary principles summarized below.

Eat three regular meals a day and include breakfast regularly. However, do not eat just because it is meal-time unless you feel you need food. Eat a variety of foods, so that you get proteins, carbohydrates, fats, minerals and vitamins. Keep the ratio of calories from protein, carbohydrate and fat close to 20%, 60% and 20% of your diet, respectively.

Fat children with a high number of fat cells usually grow into fat adults. Therefore, it is very important to introduce youngsters to nutritionally sound eating habits. Normally an average weight person with reasonably disciplined eating and exercise habits, rarely becomes obese in later life.

Maintain an ideal weight. People with normal or slightly below normal weight not only lead a healthy life but live longer than those who are overweight.

If you consume more calories than you use-whether from protein, carbohydrate, or fat-you will gain weight. The extra calories are always converted to fat and accumulate in the body as fat, no matter what their source is--a carrot or a steak or a piece of bread or a spoonful of butter. Consumption of 3,500 extra calories means a pound of body fat.

Repeated gaining, losing, and regaining of extra pounds is more damaging to your health than just remaining overweight. That is why it is important to give up the notion of a "diet." A diet is something you go on and off. Permanent weight control means an eating plan that is the same today and a year from today and for the rest of your life.

"Don't diet" is becoming the newest slogan, and a step in the right direction. Every fad diet, we know so far, is nutritionally unbalanced in one way or another, and some are downright dangerous, even if followed by healthy people for a relatively short time. Weight-loss products such as diet pills generally cause temporary water loss and do not provide a weight-loss solution. Moreover, the side effects can be very serious. The only permanent solution for weight reduction is to maintain a caloric balance by cutting food calories sensibly or by burning calories through physical activity.

To maintain proper weight and good health, consume plenty of foods such as whole-wheat bread and rolls, oatmeal, brown rice, sprouts, legumes (beans, peas, lentils), fresh fruits, vegetables, and milk and milk products (low- or no-fat). But avoid fats, oils, sugars and syrups, whole fat milk, fried foods, egg yolk, alcoholic beverages, and canned fruits with added sugars.

Unfortunately, most overweight people like the fattening foods which made them overweight in the first place. To change your habit of liking healthy foods instead of fattening foods, eat healthy foods when hungry and the fattening foods only when you are less hungry. This will help you develop a taste for healthy foods over junk foods. Although it is difficult to immediately change eating habits, with persistence you can gradually increase the amount of healthy foods over undesirable fattening and unhealthy foods.

Once you learn to live normally with food, you don't have to exercise for the sake of maintaining a normal weight. Low calorie wholesome foods will naturally help maintain caloric balance. Lack of exercise is not itself a cause of overweight. Exercise, of course, help control appetite, build body strength and burn some calories.

In general, the less fat you eat of any type, the better. But whenever possible, use vegetable oils in place of hard shortenings and animal fats. Consume healthy mono-unsaturated fats such as olive oil. For fat cravings eat nuts such as walnuts and flex seeds that provide heart healthy omega-3 fatty acids.

Limit protein intake from animal sources. Remember, only foods from animal sources are rich in cholesterol, a prime factor in coronary artery disease. In case you include animal protein, the species that are more primordial should be preferred over highly evolved ones. This means fowl such as chicken or turkey is recommended over mammal meat such as beef and pork; fish and other seafood are even more suitable than fowl. Excess protein is of no use to the body except as an energy source, in other words, calories. So you can get fat eating too much protein.

Carbohydrates are no more fattening than protein, and rough carbohydrates from whole grains, fruits and vegetables should be consumed in sufficient quantity for providing energy. The low or no carbohydrate diets such as Atkin's are gaining popularity, but these are not a solution to long-term weight problem.

It is hard to be a fat vegetarian. To reduce weight, increase the amount of vegetarian foods. With proper combinations, vegetarian foods can provide most of the necessary amino acids. In fact, vegetarian foods such as grains, roots, vegetables, and fruits in an unrefined, minimally processed form are among the best sources of protein.

Vegetarian foods provide adequate amounts of fiber, minerals, and vitamins, and are almost lacking in fat and cholesterol.

Avoid adding commercially sold fiber to your food. Use soluble fiber such as Metamucil, if you must. Good sources of fiber are fruits, vegetables, and whole grains. Sufficient addition of these foods to your daily diet should alleviate constipation and intestinal disorders. The healthy fiber known as pectin comes from natural fruits and vegetables. Pectin binds plant cells together. Guar gum that is claimed to lower cholesterol is due to its pectin component.

Vegetarians who eat no animal protein at all may require a supplement of vitamin B-12 once every several weeks. However, vegetarians who include milk and milk products in their diet get an adequate amount of vitamin B-12 from the milk and milk products.

Synthetic and natural vitamins are chemically the same and perform the same function. However, vitamins from natural foods are less concentrated and are accompanied by other nutrients which share metabolic reactions to give the full nutritional effect.

Over-cooking can destroy heat sensitive vitamins such as vitamin C, B-1 and pantothenic acid.

Too much consumption of fat soluble vitamins A, D, E, and K, may result in excessive accumulation of these vitamins in the body and thus may cause serious side effects. Excessive amounts of water soluble vitamins, B-complex and C, however, are excreted from the body. The main side effects of water soluble vitamins can be deficiency symptoms if you lower your intake from excessive amounts to normal consumption.

Milk is an excellent source of high quality protein, calcium and several other useful nutrients for children and adults. However, in people with low production of the enzyme lactase, milk sugar (lactose) cannot be broken down into glucose and galactose and can cause a problem such as an allergic reaction to undigested milk protein. So milk is a perfect food for most people, but unfortunately not for everyone. Soy milk is a healthy substitute for milk.

If possible, do not consume dairy products that are not organic because they will have growth hormone in them and will slow your weight loss. In fact, growth hormones from milk and meat is part of the reason for America's weight problem.

No diet sodas or diet food. These do not help losing weight. Sodas have been called the "new crack" because they appear to be so physically addicting. They actually make you fat. Diet foods fall into the same category. Do not eat anything that is being presented as a diet food. These do not satisfy your appetite and you end up eating more.

No white sugar or white flour. Replace white sugar with raw evaporated sugar cane juice or honey as a sweetener. In addition you can use organic molasses, organic fruit juice, organic dates, and the herb stevia. Artificial sweetners are not good for you or to control your weight. White flour with no fiber makes you eat more that makes you fat. Use whole grain flours that have not been processed or stripped of the fiber.

Eat salad. Even if you eat cheeseburger, French fries, and a pint of ice cream; add to it a big, huge salad and eat that first. The salad can contain anything you like as long as it is only vegetables. The salad dressing can be olive oil and freshly squeezed lemon juice, or vinegar. Add some sea salt, fresh ground pepper, or some garlic for taste. Don't use fatty salad dressings with cheese.

The use of salt, alcohol, and caffeine should be reduced to a minimum. Smoking is undoubtedly dangerous to health, and should obviously be avoided. No monosodium glutamate, or MSG, a flavor-enhancer. MSG is an excitotoxin. It may cause all kinds of medical problems, and can affect your mood making you depressed. It also can be physically addicting and may actually make you hungrier. Even if it is subject to further review and testing, it is better to avoid foods with MSG.

Contrary to the belief that spicy food causes stomach ulcers, it is good to add anything spicy or hot that will increase your metabolism and make you burn fat quicker. No spice is stronger than stomach acid and spicy food as a cause of ulcer is a myth.

Try to understand the nutritional values of food and-without becoming a diet freak-keep in mind the effects of various foods on your health.

You can cheat once a while, but don't feel guilty. You want ice cream, cookies, cakes, chocolate, French fries, pizza, potato chips? Don't deprive yourself. It's better to eat something without guilt than not eat something and keep thinking about it. Here's how you handle the situation from best to worst: You are offered a piece of chocolate cake. You look at it and decide that you're full and wouldn't really enjoy it, so it does not look that appealing to you. You politely say "no thanks" and feel great about your choice. You feel no depravation. This is ideal. Next would be: You are offered the chocolate cake, and you decide that you want it even though you are trying to lose weight. You say "yes" and eat the cake with happiness and glee. You enjoy and savor every bite. You're amazed at how wonderful it tastes. You are happy that you are experiencing these incredible, pleasurable sensations of this delicious cake. This is not ideal, but it is second best. Next would be a situation where you are offered the chocolate cake and you struggle with the decision. You know you are on a diet, but you can't help but imagine how wonderful this cake would taste. Inside, a voice says that nothing tastes as good as being thin feels. You struggle some more, you really want the cake, but you also want to stick to your diet. You decide to be strong and say "no." This is bad. It is better to eat the cake and enjoy it than not eat the cake and be stressed out over it. Lastly: You are offered the chocolate cake and you really want it. But you know you're on a diet and you struggle with the decision whether to indulge or be strong. You feel weak and become upset with yourself because the desire for the cake becomes overwhelming. You breakdown and eat the cake knowing full well that you shouldn't. You feel guilty and bad about yourself. This is the absolute worst. Remember: If you choose to indulge, absolutely enjoy it and be happy. Do not feel guilty or bad about it. Ideally, if you are going to cheat and eat cookies, cakes, ice cream, potato chips, etc., do not buy these products from the supermarket.

Simultaneous availability of all the necessary amino acids (units of a protein) is needed for the synthesis of a particular protein that may be required for the structure of body tissues, proper body functioning, or disease resistance. Knowledge about the combination of foods is, therefore, important to ensure an adequate supply of all the necessary amino acids. It is important to remember that people do not have to depend on meat for protein and the correct supply of amino acids. By using a proper combination, the necessary amino acids can be obtained from a vegetarian diet, thus avoiding the risks associated with higher meat consumption.

Drink a glass of water immediately upon arising. This starts the body's metabolism and cleansing. Drink eight glasses of pure water each day.

It is important to avoid overeating. Try to stop eating when you are about 80% satisfied. Occasional fasting is useful; if possible, once a month is recommended. This should be number one, but for most people this is the hardest. It is one of the fastest ways to lose weight, and one of the most effective ways to change the body's set point so that you will not gain the weight back. This should be done under supervision depending upon your medical condition.

Mastication and slow eating help to maintain a proper weight by diminishing any sensation of abnormal appetite.

The caloric intake for individuals over 50 years of age should be reduced to 90 percent of the amount required by a younger adult. In other words, a person consuming 3,000 calories would need to reduce his intake to about 2,700 calories.

Why Dieting Fails

As high as two-third of Americans are overweight, ranging from a few pounds to obese. Most of these people have been on numerous types of diets-many of which have failed.

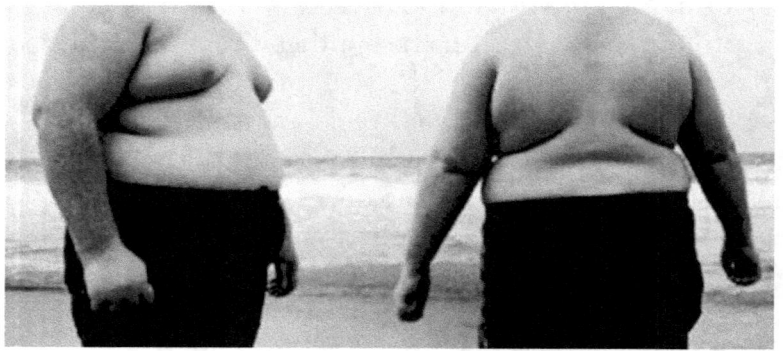

Here's why dieting no longer makes sense and new thinking about effective weight loss is the only solution, which we have presented in "A Simple Solution to America's Weight Problem".

Nature has built our bodies to survive starvation through evolutionary process. When you diet, your brain in an act of self-defense against perceived starvation signals your body that you need more food, and lowers your metabolism so you store more fat. Both actions make it harder to reach your dieting goals.

With each repeated cycle of dieting, it takes longer to lose weight and it comes back quicker. What's more, you are likely to accumulate extra pounds of fat each time.

Getting out of the diet mode requires that you accept that obesity is a complex health problem that requires a multipronged solution. Being very overweight is not simply a result of a lack of will-power or discipline, so stop blaming yourself for your size and deluding yourself that you won't wake up hungry tomorrow. You will, because your brain sabotages your best efforts at psychological control and makes it impossible to resist cravings.

Also recognize that constant dieting can perpetuate your weight problem by adversely affecting your metabolism. To keep your weight in "remission," you must be constantly vigilant, eating healthfully and exercising regularly-- is the advice most health experts give.

There are some basic weight loss facts you must keep in mind.

Low Fat Foods DON'T WORK: You cannot lose weight using Low Fat Diets. Low fat foods have been popular for decades, but yet **our society is getting more overweight as each year passes**. This fact alone should tell you that eating a purely low fat menu is not the answer to losing weight.

Low Calorie Diets DON'T WORK: You won't lose weight using a Low Calorie Dieting Plan either. In fact, eating low calories is the worst thing that you can do to your body, since that will only slow down your body's fat burning engine and ruin all chances of losing weight (low calorie diets may allow a few pounds of weight loss for the first few days, but then after that **all weight loss comes to a halt** --- known as a dieting plateau).You can never get slim by starving yourself.

Low Carb Plans DON'T WORK: You'll probably find it extremely difficult to get slim using a Low Carb Dieting Plan. Low carb diets have recently become popular over the last few years, but the problem with low carb menus is that **they are**

too strict and **TOO HARD TO FOLLOW** for **average people**. Low carb menus tend to rob your body of too much energy (carbohydrates) and make it nearly impossible to remain on the program for very long. This is why so many dieters find it difficult to follow a strict low carbohydrate menu.

What about popular dieting plans: Weight loss programs such as Weight Watchers (and Jenny Craig) usually involve slower dieting progress over a longer period of time, since

such programs generally promise only 2-3 pounds of weight loss per week. Also, programs such as Jenny Craig usually involve buying special meals and/or dietary supplements during the initial phases of the program. While some people may like these types of dietary programs, we prefer a plan that works without dieting.

A Healthy Eating Plan for Life

Here's how to start on a healthy eating plan for life.

Stop obsessing over your weight and your appetite. Rather than keeping you "in control," mental preoccupation with dieting is practically guaranteed to keep you overweight because you're constantly thinking of food.

Adhere to the following modified eating guidelines developed by the Department of Agriculture:

• Eat 20% of your calories from protein sources, 20% from fat and 60% from carbohydrates. People with a weight problem should reduce their carbohydrate intake to about 40% and increase protein intake to 40%.

• Cut back on foods that are high in saturated fats, including potato chips, ice cream and red meat. They aren't good for you and seem to spark primitive hunger urges.

• Decrease your intake of simple carbohydrates — sugars, syrups. Instead, concentrate on eating more complex carbohydrates-whole-wheat breads, rice, pasta, potatoes, fruits and vegetables-which will give you energy and make you feel full.

• Don't skip meals. Not eating at regular intervals is a foolproof way to get fat-it convinces your body you're starving and need to conserve fat.

• Don't eat less than 1,200 calories a day. When you go on such a low-calorie diet, your body starts to break down muscle tissue to use for energy so it doesn't have to dip into its fat stores. You lose weight, but you lose muscle as well as fat, which means that after your diet you'll end up with a higher percentage of body fat to muscle mass. That will make your metabolism work even slower. Remember Muscle burns fat. When you add muscle through exercise you are increasing your body's metabolism, and by losing muscle you slow metabolism.

• Start or continue an exercise program. Ideally engage in aerobic activity-walking, running, swimming or bicycling-for an hour three times a week. Second best: Exercise moderately for 30 minutes five times a week.

• To build muscle and offset muscle loss brought on by dieting, also engage in resistance training-using free weights or weight machines -twice a week. Weight training can speed your loss of fat, help you ward off osteoporosis as you age and enhance your endurance.

Remember that unless you are willing to exercise regularly, you will not succeed in keeping weight off.

It is a myth that by following a proper diet and exercise program, you can turn body fat into muscle. Fat and muscle are two separate entities. You must burn fat and build muscle.

Curious! When fat is burned, where does it actually go?

When you lose weight (by eating less and exercising more), an enzyme located in fat cells disassembles the fat compounds and sends the components into the bloodstream. Liver and muscle cells take up these components and disassemble them even further, until what's left is a compound called acetyl-CoA. Acetyl-CoA then enters the Krebs cycle, a series of chemical reactions that takes place in the mitochondria — the cell's "power plant." Krebs cycle is a part of respiration process.

The end product of this dismantling of acetyl-CoA via the Krebs cycle and subsequent cellular processes is: Carbon dioxide, which is expelled when you exhale. Water, which is lost as urine and perspiration. Heat, which helps maintain body temperature. ATP, the molecule that fuels cellular activities that require energy.

So that is how body burns fat during weight-loss and produces energy.

In addition to above suggestions, always keep small emergency snacks on hand in case you're running late for lunch or dinner — perhaps a piece of fruit, nonfat yogurt or baby carrots. You may occasionally have nuts such as walnuts and almonds for snack. The bottom line: It's about choosing an eating style that fits with your lifestyle and you can live with!

These are very sound suggestions but still not a permanent solution to weight problem. That's why *Kapalbhati*, a main technique in this book, is finally a successful way to go.

2

Weight Maintenance

The hard part isn't losing weight, but keeping it off. Despite the best nutrition, exercise regimens and diet plans in the world, 90% of dieters regain one- to two-thirds of lost weight within one year and almost all of it within five years. Because they are not able to eat frozen dinners and drink low-cal shakes for the rest of their life, that is almost impossible on most of the commercial weight-loss programs. Each year, Americans spend $33 billion on commercial diet programs-and much of that sum is essentially wasted.

Not surprising, then, that many dieters shuffle unsuccessfully from one diet plan to the next-losing weight on one program, putting it back on and then moving on to another plan.

In fact, counselors working for the leading commercial diet plans freely admit that perhaps nine of 10 people who try one commercial diet program wind up trying two or three or more.

It's a lot easier to lose weight than it is to keep off the excess pounds. When you are trying to lose weight, you're singularly focused on the task at hand. But once you're down to your target weight, you have to balance weight maintenance with other factors in your life.

On a daily basis, that requires you to continually correct yourself and bring yourself back on course.

Weight management is a journey rather than a destination.

Psychology of Weight Maintenance

Why is it so hard to lose weight and keep it off? It is not because we don't know which foods to eat and which to avoid.

In most cases, persistent obesity is the result of irrational beliefs, which make us using food to satisfy emotional, not physical, hunger.

By replacing these beliefs with sound self-statements, it's possible to change our eating behavior-and our weight.

Start with Self-Acceptance: Few people recognize the incredible irony that underlies most cases of obesity-that is, if you're serious about losing weight, you must first learn to accept yourself. You must do so unconditionally, with all your eating and weight problems.

Putting yourself down-for being fat, for falling short of your eating goals or for any other reason-may feel like a powerful motivational tool. In fact, it hampers your efforts to change your eating habits.

If you habitually put yourself down, you'll eventually come to view yourself as weak and unable to change-and, perhaps, not worth changing.

Self-flagellation also makes you feel bad. And people regularly use overeating to soothe bad feelings.

How does one move toward greater self-acceptance? There are two key strategies:

Focus on behavior. Don't confuse what you do with who you are. Just because you overeat (behavior) does not mean you're a bad person (character).

Each of us does millions of things during a lifetime. Some are good. Some are bad. Learn to say, "Overeating is bad" rather than, "1 am bad."

Change "should" and "must" to preferences. Should and must are among the most common-and most destructive-irrational beliefs. "if you think that...

• Life should be less stressful...

• You should be able to eat whatever you want...

• You must become thinner...

• Other people must treat you fairly...

...then you'll feel angry and miserable when these demands aren't met.

Let's face it. Life isn't fair, and others don't always treat us the way we'd like them to. Yet insisting that things be otherwise doesn't change things. It just wastes time and energy and makes us chronically upset.

When we recast these demands as preferences, they lose their power to make us miserable.

For example: Don't tell yourself, "I must be thin." Tell yourself, "I prefer to be thin."

In conclusion: Positive thinking patterns are crucial to successful, long-term weight management.

People who are not successful at managing their weight tend to:

• Make excuses that let them overeat or not exercise.

• Focus narrowly on the pleasure of eating and forget their weight-management goals.

•Doubt their ability to change.

•Set unrealistic expectations for themselves or others.

•Judge themselves-and other people-harshly.

In contrast, those people who are successful tend to:

•Remind themselves of their long-range goals.

•Notice even small successes in weight management.

•Use positive self-talk to keep themselves on the right track.

Strategies for Weight Maintenance

• **Exercise.** You've heard it over and over again, but exercise is truly the key to weight -control success. **Make exercise a regular part of your life.** Without regular exercise, weight maintenance is exceedingly difficult. The more you exercise the more muscle you build. And because muscle cells burn dietary fat more efficiently than fat cells do, gaining muscle mass speeds your metabolism. Thus a thin person can eat much more fat than a fat person without gaining weight.

Of course, making exercise a part of your daily routine is easier said than done. Choose a range of activities that you enjoy. The point is to do what you like. Otherwise, you'll quickly give up exercising. If you used to play a lot of volleyball or softball, for example, try to work these activities back into your schedule. If you're joining a gym, look for one where you feel comfortable. One reason people stop going to the gym is that they feel they don't measure up. If you feel intimidated by a fancy club, try the local "Y" instead.

In fact you don't need any gym, walk outside for an hour a day. The body is designed to walk. Research shows that slow, rhythmic movement exercise, such as walking, resets your body's weight set point and creates a thin, lean body. A one-hour walk everyday will change your body dramatically in as little as one month. On days when it rains, cycle on a stationary bicycle indoors.

Build exercise into your everyday life: climb the stairs instead of taking the escalator. Walk to the corner store instead of taking the car. Park far away from the mall so you'll have farther to walk. These are just few examples. You can add many more to this list.

• **Reduce fat calories** to 20% of your daily intake. Most Americans eat more fat than they need. We're exposed to a lot of fatty, highly palatable foods, so we develop a taste for foods that are readily available. However, you can change your taste buds and actually learn to prefer low-fat foods. But make a gradual change because you're changing the way you eat for the rest of your life. Eat bread without butter, salad with little or no dressing and chicken without its skin. Start by switching to milk instead of cream in your coffee, drink low fat or even better no fat milk, then switching to low-fat mayonnaise on your sandwiches, etc.

Eat what you like. If you already enjoy certain low-fat foods, make them staples of your diet. Make a list of your favorite high-fat foods, and find a way to substitute low-fat versions for some of them. Also when eating a meal containing high-fat food, eat a small amount of that food and balance it with low-fat choices-lots of vegetables, or fruit for dessert.

After consuming low-fat foods for a while, you'll find that eating fatty foods makes you feel physically and psychologically uncomfortable-- bloated, sluggish, even nauseous.

Use "fat banking" to maintain a healthful diet without feeling as if you can never have fatty foods. Look at calorie and fat allotments as balances in a bank account. You can draw on them as you would from a bank. If you know you will want a high-fat food on a certain day, you can "build up your bank balance" by cutting your fat intake for some days before- or reducing fat intake afterward to bring your account back into balance.

• **Control binges.** Between 25% and 50% of all people who attend weight-management programs are bingers. The biggest trigger for binges is negative emotions: anger, depression, anxiety.

Keep a two-week journal to record your eating behaviors-meals, snacks, binges. Also record the circumstances-how you feel, what you are doing and your thoughts when you are eating. This will help you identify triggers for eating and develop strategies to avoid them.

• **Eat moderately.** To successfully maintain a low weight level, you must keep your caloric intake under control.

Eat anything you want, but keep your calories in a moderate range. The government recommends between 1,600 and 2,800 calories each day to maintain weight for most adult men and women. However, your best range for maintaining weight will depend on your age, sex, lifestyle, activity level and other factors. Experiment with adding on and taking off calories to find the range that's best for you.

• **Do not eat after seven in the evening.** Do the best you can on this. However, you can eat all day long. And if you stop eating after 7:00 p.m., you will reduce the calories accumulating as fat at night.

• **Think smart.** Focus on your long-term goal of weight maintenance, give yourself instructional thoughts and pat yourself on the back for positive behaviors.

• **Control stress.** When you are under pressure, your body produces cortisol-a hormone that tells your body to put out more neuropeptides and galanin. As a result, you crave carbohydrates and fats. The research has supported that stressed people end up being obese. A new kind of product

being touted is cortisol-control aids, such as Relacore and CortiSlim, which promise to banish the spare tire around your middle by reducing your levels of this "stress hormone." But the ultimate solution is to use stress-busters.

While you can't eliminate stress entirely, you can learn to control it. Find the best stress-buster for you-exercise, practice deep breathing or meditation, perform muscle relax-and-release exercises, take a warm bath, read a book, or listen to music. **"Art of Stress-free Living"** by Dr. S.S. Dhillon is a good start to handle stress.

For some people, stress reduction actually suppresses the appetite by decreasing levels of certain compounds in the body that can spur weight gain.

Eating is often a survival skill. It's a way of coping with frustrations and disappointments. Life can be very difficult. Eating can get you through it.

Overeating becomes a way to maintain emotional health-although physical health is jeopardized as a result.

To overcome this self-destructive approach to food, you must learn to separate food itself from its emotional symbolism.

• **Get enough sleep.** Strange but true. During sleep, not only our bodies rest and regenerate, but sleep is important component of weight control. Sleep deprivation causes an imbalance in certain hormones, including ghrelin (which causes weight gain) and leptin (which decreases appetite). When we don't get enough sleep, our levels of ghrelin go up (more weight gain) and levels of leptin go down (so we are hungrier). Don't think of it as downtime, but as another important facet of your nutrition plan.

• **Handle lapses.** Everyone backslides on occasion. Avoid turning a lapse into a relapse. Instead of having a second donut, go out for a walk or go to the gym to burn off the calories or cut back on calorie intake tomorrow.

• **Accept your body**. Focus not on how your body looks, but on what it enables you to do. Don't compare yourself with the ideal body put forth in sexy movies or magazine ads. After all, body shape is determined largely by heredity. We tend to look like our mothers and fathers-and that persists even if we're successful at losing weight.

• **Make food a pleasure.** Avoid thinking of food as a moral issue. "Good" foods are those you think you should be eating: fruits, vegetables, beans, wholegrain breads, etc. "Bad" foods taste good but are fattening: cakes, candy, sugary soft drinks, etc.

Substituting good foods for bad sounds like a good idea, but odds are it's just setting you up for failure. Because even if you could steer clear of "bad" foods for several months, you'd give in to temptation-possibly by going on an eating binge.

Therefore, if you like cheesecake, allow yourself the freedom to eat it on occasion. By removing this cheesecake "taboo," you reduce your obsession with it.

• **Create a lifestyle that is satisfying to you.** The last thing you want to say at the end of your life is that you devoted the majority of your life to watching your weight. While weight maintenance is important to health and psychological well-being, your life should be about something more meaningful.

Create a mission that makes you feel your life is worth living. Find a way to be creative, contribute to society or do something that's important to you.

• There is no end to strange expert advices. To lose weight via **"scent therapy,"** try these simple strategies, suggests Dr. Alan R. Hirsch, MD, Rush-Presbyterian-St. Luke's Medical Center in Chicago.

• Take time to sniff your food before eating. Inhale as deeply as possible to make sure the aroma-causing molecules reach the olfactory bulb. That's the part of the body responsible for the sense of smell .

• Chew your food thoroughly. The more thoroughly you chew, the more scent is liberated. If you're eating alone-or can do so without offending your dining partner-you might even try "blowing bubbles" into each mouthful of food before swallowing. By doing so, you maximize the mixing of food molecules with air molecules. (I wouldn't dare to try blowing bubbles and swallowing air into my stomach whether alone or in a company.)

• Opt for fresh foods whenever possible- and eat them hot. Fresh, unprocessed foods tend to have stronger scents than packaged or canned foods. Hot food is more aromatic than cold food.

• Add a pungent herb, spice or condiment to bland foods. If you're eating rice, for example, you might top it with steak sauce. You might sprinkle chopped garlic on your salad ... or add a splash of ketchup on cottage cheese.

With all the expert advice, make it a habit to follow *kapalbhati* which has worked for me and many others, and there is no substitute for its effectiveness. It can be done anywhere, at any age and with any level of physical fitness.

Specific Hints to Keep Weight Off

• **Surprising Calorie-Burner:** Sipping ice water burns calories. Whenever you drink something cold, your body raises your metabolism to keep your body temperature from falling. That process burns calories: eight 16-ounce glasses of ice water will burn an extra 200 calories per day.

Keeping low heat in winter will also help burn extra calories and will save you on energy bill.

• **Dieting vs. Your Set Point:** The only way to ensure lasting weight loss is to lower your set point-the weight your body "thinks" it should weigh. When people overeat, they generally gain weight only temporarily, returning to their usual weight, or "set point" when they resume their previous eating habits.

Similarly, when you go on a low-calorie diet, your body wants to keep you from starving. As a result, your metabolism slows to maintain your set point. Therefore, weight loss occurs very slowly. When you resume your normal eating patterns, your weight quickly rises to its former level.

To lower your set point, reduce your intake of dietary fat and increase your lean muscle mass. In other words, lighten up your eating habits and exercise enough to build muscle.

• **Metabolism Slows With Age:** Metabolism slows with age-beginning as early as age 35. Therefore, you gain weight simply from continuing to eat as you did when you were younger.

However, it is a myth that there is nothing you can do about that. While it's true our metabolism naturally slows down by about 2-5% per decade after age 40, there are plenty of things we can do to fight back.

Exercise is key. Engage in aerobic exercise 4 to 5 days a week: It's obvious that aerobic activities like running, brisk walking, breathing exercises, swimming and bike riding burn calories and increase metabolism while you're working out. But interestingly enough, several studies show that aerobic activities cause your metabolism to stay increased for a period of time after exercising.

Work your muscles: Lifting weights and/or other strengthening activities like push-ups and crunches on a regular basis (at least 2-3 times each week) will boost your resting metabolism 24/7. That's because these activities build muscle, and muscle burns more calories than body fat. In fact, if you have more muscle, you burn more calories — even sitting still.

When it comes to food, keep your metabolism revved with these three tips:

1. Eat enough food — at least 1000 calories: Your body and metabolism thrive on food; when you fast, crash-diet or restrict calories below 1000, your metabolism will SLOW down in a response to conserve energy.

2. Eat every 4-5 hours: Because our bodies work hard to digest and absorb the foods we eat, your metabolism revs in response. This is called the thermic effect of food. Take full advantage and schedule meals and snacks every 4-5 hours.

3. Incorporate lean protein with every meal: Eating all foods creates a thermic effect and will boost metabolism after consumption. However, the consumption of protein has the absolute greatest metabolic boost when compared to carbohydrate and fat. PLUS, eating the appropriate amount of protein will ensure you're able to maintain and build muscle mass (the more muscle mass you have, the greater your metabolism).

Daily Protein Requirements: 50% of your weight = daily grams of protein

Some of the best protein sources include: fish, chicken, turkey, lean sirloin steak, skim milk, yogurt, eggs and egg substitutes, tofu and beans. Egg-white, normally from boiled egg, is my preferred source of protein.

In conclusion: to keep up with age-related metabolic decline, weight training and regular aerobic exercise will increase muscle mass and keep your metabolism running more quickly. Also, consume foods that are full of nutrients but low in calories-drink vegetable juice instead of soda, eat multigrain bread instead of white. You can continue eating most of your favorite foods-just reduce the portion sizes.

NOTE: To keep up exercise and to increase muscle mass with age is doable but not easy for most of the people and puts lot of burden on the body and skeleton. That's why it is easy said than done. It again comes down to our special techniques described in this book that can be done at any age.

Overweight Concerns at Various Ages

Since calorie requirements change with age, appropriate eating habits at various ages is important to maintain a proper weight throughout your life. Here's what you need to keep in mind.

Infants (under 2 year): Breast-feeding supplies infants with needed nutrients in just the right amounts (in addition to providing antibodies for fighting infections). Bottle-feeding with formulas often turns out heavier babies, which leads to obesity in later life.

Children (2 to 12 years): At this stage, we develop lifelong habits of eating and exercise. Limit TV-watching; and promote lots of physical activity--cycling, skating, swimming, climbing etc. Serve low-fat, high-carbohydrate, good protein foods.

Teenagers (13 to 19 years): More than weight, the concern is to build bones and muscle through this growth phase. Pay particular attention to include foods like four or more glasses of skim milk, beans, whole-grain breads, potatoes, lean meats, dried fruits, and other low-fat but nutritious foods.

Young Adults (20 to 39 years): If you build a foundation of good eating habits in your childhood and teen years, you probably can coast on it up to age 40. For those of you who once played active sports and who now take your sports via TV, flab begins to replace muscle. This may be your last chance to control weight easily by adopting eating and exercise patterns for a lifetime.

Middle-aged (40 to 60 years): For most of us, our body weight creeps up between ages 40 and 60, initiating "middle-aged spread." Our metabolism (the process by which our bodies burn energy) slows down, so our bodies are burning fewer calories. Much of that extra weight also comes from less activity and taking in more high-fat foods and alcohol.

Seniors (61 to 80 years): After age 60 and before 80, food problems multiply. Pay attention to increasing calcium intake and lowering sodium intake. Keep down intake of animal fats and keep up your intake of rough carbohydrates.

Over 80-years: Diet becomes even more important. Minor changes in diet can lead to substantial improvements. High-fiber foods can clear up much digestive discomfort, including constipation. In addition to increasing minerals, vitamins and fiber, keep down intake of animal fat and keep up intake of rough carbohydrates.

3

Kids and Teenage Weight Problem

Kids and teenage weight problem has become a serious concern not only in terms of looks but major health, psychological, and even social issue. The research findings are quite alarming.

Juvenile Obesity and Its Consequences

High Blood Pressure: The findings reported by Reuters August 21, 2007, have shown that high blood pressure among children and adolescents, is a growing problem linked to increasing juvenile obesity. It often goes undiagnosed in the United States despite doctors' visits because it is normally a disease of adults and old. It is a serious concern, as high blood pressure can quietly damage the organs, especially the kidneys, the researchers reported in August-2007 Journal of the American Medical Association. High blood pressure, or hypertension, often signals another disease in children, like endocrine disorders, kidney or heart disease.

Researchers at Case Western Reserve University in Cleveland examined more than 14,000 young people ages 3 to 18 and found 507 cases of hypertension. Nearly three quarters of that group, or 376 cases, had not been diagnosed despite at least three previous medical checkups.

An estimated 3.6 percent of the children had high blood pressure, within the range found in other studies, according to Dr. Matthew Hansen and colleagues.

They suggested that electronic medical recordkeeping could be upgraded to better diagnose the problem by comparing the findings of earlier checkups, even though juvenile hypertension is difficult to confirm because it varies by sex, height and weight.

"Identification of elevated blood pressure in children meeting prehypertension or hypertension criteria is important because of the increasing prevalence of pediatric weight problems," the researchers wrote.

"If abnormal blood pressure is not identified by a patient's pediatric clinician, it may be years before the abnormal blood pressure is detected, leading to end-organ damage," they added.

Obese children miss more school: Obesity not only effects physical health, but obese elementary schoolchildren miss a couple more school days on average than their normal-weight classmates, according to a study that says being fat is a better predictor for absenteeism than any other factor.

Researchers said their results suggest that childhood obesity, in addition to serious medical issues, can lead to a plethora of additional problems down the road.

"It's clear in all the literature that the more days of school you miss, it really sets you up for such negative outcomes: drugs and AIDS and (teen) pregnancy," said Andrew B. Geier, a doctoral candidate at the University of Pennsylvania and lead author of the study.

He said the findings should serve as a clarion call to school officials.

"At this early age to show that already they're missing school, and missing school is such a major setup for big-time problems, that's something school policy people have to know," Geier said.

Obesity is found to be the bigger cause of absenteeism than gender or race. The researchers from Penn and Temple University looked at 1,069 fourth- to sixth-graders for one academic year in nine Philadelphia schools, where teachers took attendance each morning. Based on body mass index, a standard measure of height and weight, each child was classified as underweight, normal weight, overweight or obese.

Of 180 school days, researchers found that on average the normal weight students missed 10.1 days, overweight kids missed 10.9 days and obese children missed 12.2 days. For reasons that aren't clear, underweight children had the fewest absences — 7.5 on average.

In decades of research about student performance, race, socioeconomic status, age and gender have been tagged as the top predictors for absenteeism. The new study, in the August-2007 issue of the journal Obesity, concludes that weight tops them all, Geier said.

The study didn't explore why the children missed school. Researchers theorize it's got less to do with medical issues — many children at this young age haven't yet developed major obesity-linked maladies — and more to do with the stigma of being fat.

"They're missing school because they don't want to be bullied and called names," Geier said.

Researchers tried to make the test group as homogeneous as possible by picking schools that were among the city's poorest, with the assumption that education and income levels would be fairly even.

Nationally, obesity rates have nearly quintupled among 6- to 11-year-olds and tripled among teens and children ages 2 to 5 since the 1970s, according to the Centers for Disease Control and Prevention. Obesity can lead to diabetes, high blood pressure and cholesterol, sleep apnea and orthopedic problems.

The study adds to growing research into non-medical complications of being fat, including data suggesting that obese adults miss more workdays and go to college less frequently than people of normal weight, Geier said.

"This is exactly the kind of study that will get the attention of policy makers," said Jim Bogden, healthy eating project coordinator for the National Association of State Boards of Education. "The correlation with absenteeism is very powerful."

Overweight kids face widespread stigma from rejection to suicide: Overweight children are stigmatized by their peers as early as age 3 and even face bias from their parents and teachers, giving them a quality of life comparable to people with cancer, a new analysis concludes.

Youngsters who report teasing, rejection, bullying and other types of abuse because of their weight are two to three times more likely to report suicidal thoughts as well as to suffer from other health issues such as high blood pressure and eating disorders, researchers said.

"The stigmatization directed at obese children by their peers, parents, educators and others is pervasive and often unrelenting," researchers with Yale University and the University of Hawaii at Manatoa wrote in the July-2007 issue of Psychological Bulletin.

The paper was based on a review of all research on youth weight bias over the past 40 years, said lead author Rebecca M. Puhl of Yale's Rudd Center for Food Policy and Obesity.

It comes amid a growing worldwide epidemic of child obesity. By 2010, almost 50 percent of children in North America and 38 percent of children in the European Union will be overweight, the researchers said.

While programs to prevent childhood obesity are growing, more efforts are needed to protect overweight children from abuse, Puhl said.

"The quality of life for kids who are obese is comparable to the quality of life of kids who have cancer," Puhl said, citing one study. "These kids are facing stigma from everywhere they look in society, whether it's media, school or at home."

Even with a growing percentage of overweight people, the stigma shows no signs of subsiding, according to Puhl. She said television and other media continue to reinforce negative stereotypes.

"This is a form of bias that is very socially acceptable," Puhl said. "It is rarely challenged; it's often ignored."

The stigmatization of overweight children has been documented for decades. When children were asked to rank photos of children as friends in a 1961 study, the overweight child was ranked last.

Children as young as 3 are more likely to consider overweight peers to be mean, stupid, ugly and sloppy.

A growing body of research shows that parents and educators are also biased against heavy children. In a 1999 study of 115 middle and high school teachers, 20 percent said they believed obese people are untidy, less likely to succeed and more emotional.

"Perhaps the most surprising source of weight stigma toward youths is parents," the report says.

Several studies showed that overweight girls got less college financial support from their parents than average weight girls. Other studies showed teasing by parents was common.

"It is possible that parents may take out their frustration, anger and guilt on their overweight child by adopting stigmatizing attitudes and behavior, such as making critical and negative comments toward their child," the authors wrote, suggesting further research is needed.

Lynn McAfee, 58, of Stowe, Pa., said that as an overweight child she faced troubles on all fronts. "It was constantly impressed upon me that I wasn't going to get anywhere in the world if I was fat," McAfee said. "You hear it so often, it becomes the truth."

Her mother, who also was overweight, offered to buy her a mink coat when she was 8 to try to get her to lose weight even though her family was poor. "I felt I was letting everybody down," she said.

Other children would try to run her down on bikes to see if she would bounce. She had a hard time getting on teams in the playground.

"Teachers did not stand up for me when I was teased," McAfee said.

A study in 2003 found that obese children had much lower quality of life scores on issues such as health, emotional and social well-being, and school functioning.

Sylvia Rimm, author of "Rescuing the Emotional Lives of Overweight Children," said her surveys of more than 5,000 middle school children reached similar conclusions.

"The overweight children felt less intelligent," Rimm said. "They felt less popular. They struggled from early on. They feel they are a different species."

Parents should emphasize a child's strengths, she said, and teachers should pair up students for activities instead of letting children pick their partners.

McAfee, who now works for the Council on Size and Weight Discrimination, said her childhood experiences even made her reluctant to see a doctor when she needed one. She recalled one doctor who said she looked like a gorilla and another who gave her painkillers and diet pills for what turned out to be mononucleosis.

"The amount of cruelty I've seen in people has changed me forever," McAfee said.

"Weight-based discrimination is as important a problem as racial discrimination or discrimination against children with physical disabilities," the report concludes. "Remedying it needs to be taken equally seriously..."

Why Diet Foods Don't Work

The diet foods, not only don't work but instead might cause kids to overeat. The diet sodas and snacks so popular with weight-conscious adults may backfire in children, if new animal research is correct.

In experiments with juvenile rats, researchers at the University of Alberta in Canada found that animals that became used to diet foods tended to overeat during meals of regular-calorie animal chow. This was true for normal-weight and obese rat pups, the researchers found. However, diet foods did not appear to have an overeating effect in adolescent rats.

This suggests that the foods have some unique effect in young animals, and possibly children, the study authors report in the August-2007 journal Obesity.

They suspect that diet foods disrupted the young animals' ability to learn how various flavors correlate with calories.

When they associate tastes, such as sweet or salty, with few calories, even a rich dessert may fail to fill them up as it otherwise would.

It's possible that children given artificially low-calorie snacks and diet sodas might not learn to properly regulate their food intake, according to lead study author Dr. W. David Pierce.

"One thing is clear at this point," he said in a statement. "Young animals and perhaps children can be made to overeat when calorie-wise foods are offered on a daily basis, subverting the body's energy-balance system."

He and his colleagues recommend that parents give their children a well-balanced diet of foods in their natural form, including naturally low-calorie foods like fruits and vegetables.

The findings are based on a series of experiments with young rats, both normal, lean animals and those genetically prone to obesity. Over 16 days, the animals were regularly given gelatin cubes that contained starch, as well as a starch-free "diet" version of the snack.

For some animals, the starchy cubes were flavored with an artificial sweetener and the diet version was flavored with a salty solution. These flavors were reversed for other animals.

After 16 days of this taste training, the researchers gave all the animals a high-calorie snack dipped in either artificial sweetener or a salty solution. They then gave the rats a meal of their regular chow.

Pierce's team found that the animals tended to overeat during the meal if their pre-meal snack had been dipped in a flavor they'd learn to associate with a low-calorie food — despite the snack's actual high calorie content.

The phenomenon was seen in both lean and obesity-prone rat pups, but the heavier animals generally ate more than their normal-weight counterparts, the researchers point out.

So it's possible, they say, that diet foods could be especially detrimental in the children already at the greatest risk of long-term weight problems.

Diet food fads have not helped adults either, as evident from overweight statistics. In conclusion, diet foods are not a solution to lose weight.

What's Wrong with Nutrition Education!

The federal government will spend more than $1 billion this year on nutrition education — fresh carrot and celery snacks, videos of dancing fruit, hundreds of hours of lively lessons about how great you will feel if you eat well.

But an Associated Press review of dozens of rigorous scientific studies shows that these programs almost never change the way kids eat. And there is no indication they will make a dent in the growing epidemic of childhood obesity.

"Any person looking at the published literature about these programs would have to conclude that they are generally not working," said Dr. Tom Baranowski, a pediatrics professor at Houston's Baylor College of Medicine who studies behavioral nutrition.

The evidence is in the children. Nationally, obesity rates have nearly quintupled among 6- to 11-year-olds and tripled among teens and children ages 2 to 5 since the 1970s, according to the Centers for Disease Control. The medical consequences of obesity in the U.S. — diabetes, high blood pressure, even orthopedic problems — cost an estimated $100 billion a year. Kentucky cardiologist Dr. James W. Holsinger

Jr., nominated as the surgeon general, says fighting childhood obesity is his top priority. So does the first lady Michelle Obama in 2010. Thus far, the federal government had put its money on education as the solution. But a review of 57 trials aimed at changing kids' eating habits found just four showed any real success.

These observation reinforce the disappointing studies:

In 2006 a major federal pilot program offering free fruits and vegetables to school children showed fifth graders became less willing to eat them than they had at the start. Apparently they didn't like the taste.

In Pennsylvania, researchers went so far as to give prizes to school children who ate fruits and vegetables. That worked while the prizes were offered, but when the researchers came back seven months later the kids had reverted to their original eating habits: soda and chips.

In studies where children tell researchers they are eating better or exercising more, there is usually no change in blood pressure, body size or cholesterol measures; they want to eat better, they might even think they are, but they're not.

So far nutrition programs has become a losing battle against obesity. The studies don't tell Leticia Jenkins anything she doesn't know. She's one of the concerned teachers in America — not because she gave her seventh and eighth graders 30

sharp knives to chop tomatoes, onions, jalapenos and limes for a lesson on salsa and nutrition, but because she understands the futility of what she is trying to do.

"Oh, it's so hard, because at the end of the day sometimes I take a moment, I think gosh, I did all this and we still see them across the street picking up the doughnuts and the coffee drinks," she said.

The challenges to changing the way children eat are as numerous as the factors that have prompted the obesity epidemic in the first place.

The forces that make kids fat "are really strong and hard to fight with just a program in school," said Dr. Philip Zeitler, a pediatric endocrinologist and researcher who sees "a steady stream" of obese children struggling with diabetes and other potentially fatal medical problems at The Children's Hospital in Denver.

What does he tell them? "Oh God, I haven't figured out anything that I know is going to work," he said. "I'm not aware of any medical model that is very successful in helping these kids. Sure, we try to help them, but I can't take credit for the ones who do manage to change."

The obstacles are daunting:

Parental influence is lot more important than any of school or other programs. Experts agree that although most funding targets schools, parents have the greatest influence, even a biological influence, over what their children will eat. When children slim down, it's mostly because "the families have figured out what needs to happen." But often, they don't.

Obesity often runs in families. "If the mother is eating Cheetos and white bread, the fetus will be born with those taste buds. If the mother is eating carrots and oatmeal the child will be born with those taste buds," said Dr. Robert Trevino, at the Social and Health Research Center in San Antonio, Texas.

Most kids learn what tastes good and what tastes nasty by their 10th birthdays.

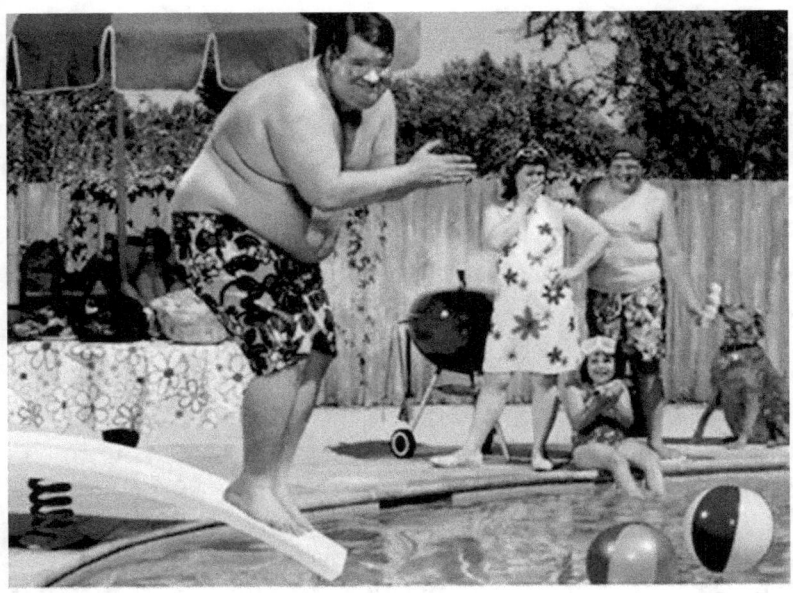

"If we don't reach a child before they get to puberty, it's going to be very tough, very difficult, to change their eating behavior," said Trevino.

May not always be true, but poorer kids are especially at risk because unhealthy food is cheaper and more easily available than healthy food. Parents are often working, leaving children unsupervised to get their own snacks. Low-income neighborhoods have fewer good supermarkets with fresh produce.

"If Mom can't find tomatoes in her local grocery store, nothing is going to change," said Zeitler.

Burning calories is also harder for poor children to exercise on their own. Parks often aren't safe or don't exist in close vicinity and sports teams cost money.

"Calorie burning has become the province of the wealthy," said Zeitler. "I fear that what we're going to see is a divergence of healthy people and unhealthy people. Basically, like everything else, it costs money to be healthy."

In contrast to what Zeitler and many others says that obesity is related to financial situation. Wholesome simple food is cheaper if parents are willing to spend time in preparation whether rich or poor. If parents go out for a walk, children will do that too. And no parks or expensive gym are needed to control weight. Yes, money does help to make thing easier but parental life style and commitment is more important. Slim adults are likely to have slim kids

Lure of advertisers add fuel to the fire. Children between 8 and 12 see an average of 21 television ads each day for candy, snacks, cereal and fast food — more than 7,600 a year, according to a recent Kaiser Family Foundation study. Not one of the 8,854 ads reviewed promoted fruits or vegetables.

Thinking or learning about nutrition education without practicing it is not going to do anything unless it brings changes. George Rico, a 13-year-old whose mother is a manager at a local McDonald's, said he loves his nutrition class. But does it affect what he puts in his mouth?

"Well, no, but it makes me think about what I eat," he said. "I think kids don't change because they've been eating it for so long they're just accustomed to eating that way." Their teacher, Jenkins, offers fact-filled and engaging nutrition lessons as part of a $7 million USDA program which reaches about 388,000 students a year in the Los Angeles Unified School District.

The most recent evaluation of the 8-year-old program was disheartening: No difference in the amount of fruits and vegetables eaten by kids participating in the program and those who weren't. Teachers who spent more hours on nutrition education had no greater impact than those who didn't. And parent behavior didn't change either.

"It's true, it didn't change what they actually eat. But the program really made a difference in how kids were feeling about fruits and vegetables. They really had a more positive attitude toward fruits and vegetables," said Dr. Mike Prelip, a UCLA researcher who headed up the evaluation.

Kate Houston, the deputy under secretary of the USDA's Food, Nutrition and Consumer Services, oversees most federal funds, $696 million this year, spent on childhood nutrition education in this country. Funding has steadily increased in recent years, up from $535 million in 2003. Houston insists the programs are successful. "I think the question here is how are we measuring success and there are certainly many ways in which you can do so and the ways in which we've been able to measure have shown success," she said.

But isn't the goal of these programs to change the way kids eat?

"Absolutely that's the goal," she said.

And they're successfully reaching that goal?

"We're finding success in things in which we have been able to measure, which are more related to knowledge and skill. It is more difficult for us to identify success in changing children's eating patterns."

When asked about the many studies that don't show improvement, Houston asked for copies of the research. And she said the USDA doesn't have the resources to undertake "long term, controlled, medical modeled studies" necessary to determine the impact of its programs.

Focusing on behavior, not just education about nutrition is important. Doctors like Tom Robinson, who directs the Center for Healthy Weight at Lucile Packard Children's Hospital at Stanford University, said nutrition education studies aren't needed. The research has already shown they don't work.

"I think the money could be better spent on programs that are more behaviorally oriented, as opposed to those that are educationally oriented, or studies that just describe the problem over and over again," he said.

There may be pieces of solutions found in limited studies currently being tested around the country. In some situations, obese and overweight children can lose weight and get healthy through rigorous hospital and clinic-based interventions that involve regular check-ins, family involvement, scheduled exercise and nutrition education.

School programs that increase physical activity are also more likely to have an impact than nutrition education.

This spring the Robert Wood Johnson Foundation announced plans to spend $500 million over the next five years to reverse the trend of childhood obesity. It will fund programs that bring supermarkets into poor neighborhoods, studies that measure the weight of children who exercise more at school, meetings of advocates who seek to restrict junk food ads. One thing it won't fund: projects that only provide school nutrition education.

In conclusion unless the parents take responsibility, nutrition education is not going to create slimmer kids. Only slimmer parents are likely to create slimmer kids.

How to Teach Your Kids to Eat Healthy

Childhood obesity is on the rise. How do you teach your kids healthy eating habits? What has worked for you? Here are some views, expressed over the internet by the parents.

1. Eat healthy yourself. Don't be overweight. Share vegetables with them with a smiling face of course when they are very small. Enjoy apples more than ice cream. You teach them by eating healthy yourself and cooking healthy at home. Find an overweight child, and 90% of the time you'll find overweight parents. Find a thin child, and 90% of the time you'll find thin parents. Kids don't do as you say, they do as you do.

Feed your kids what you eat and don't prepare a separate 'kids meal'. Enjoy the benefits of a well timed piece of chocolate, like once a week! You can make a 2-year old kid to have broccoli, tomatoes, and keep coming to the fruit drawer in the fridge, if you keep them unfamiliar with candy and chicken fingers!

Juice vegetables as a breakfast, or supplement to breakfast. It's not the most wonderful taste, but, the alkaline content will offset much of the acidic foods commonly consumed by children, and adults, alike. This is a fantastic health benefit that is avoided in our diets.

2. In addition to healthy foods, smaller portions at meals will keep fat content, and cholesterol, in check. Americans should take a long, hard look at the Dutch way of life: small portion meals and plenty of activity such as bicycling. Anyone who has been to The Netherlands can testify that their citizens are healthy, lean, and happy.

3. There are many issues about obesity and unhealthy eating and one we don't hear mentioned is that because produce is

picked before ripening it has a lousy taste when you buy it and is not tempting to eat. Taste is very important and that is why food companies focus on taste when hook kids to the snacks.

Try taking kids to a field when the produce is picked ripe it has a wonderful flavor whether fruits or vegetables. Kids love to go out and pick and eat blueberries, the corn that come from the local farm and the different veggies from the garden.

Maybe we should think more of community gardens especially in poor areas and getting meat, dairy and vegetables more inexpensively to the poor.

4. You hear people saying "I'm on a strict budget and what is cheap and filling is usually the unhealthy foods." This excuse has been used many times by consumers and experts alike, but it is a fact that prepared unhealthy foods are far more expensive on a per serving basis than purchasing meat and veggies and cooking yourself... do a bit more research and you will find that the above statement is erroneous!

5. When they are older, play tag. Run. Treasure outdoor activities together but end the activities before you are both exhausted. It makes them want more.

Encourage Sports along with reading. Encourage anything that get children moving. It can be a roller skating summer camp or Scuba diving on the North coast.

As always, a gym membership is recommended, especially for the youth. Even two days a week results in over 100 days per year workout.

6. Some folks in ages 60s and over may have grown up at a time when, "go outside and play" were the watchwords of mothers everywhere. No, it wasn't "quality" time with the

kids, but it was time when kids climb trees, ride bikes, make "snow forts", and so on. Lots of outlets for kid energy which translated to weight control. With all the physical activity and consumption of unprocessed, unpreserved foods, perhaps more youngsters were under weight rather than over weight.

We wish kids today had the time/chance to swing like Tarzan from a rope swing into a lake, slide down a haymow, toboggan down a long hill, build a "fort", run around the outside of the house playing.

Weight problems today with kids are so much deeper than "education"; it requires an entire change in the way we live to make lasting differences.

It's adults who gives, a kid too young to know about health, the cash for candy and pop at school or home.

7. Many times it isn't about the food. It is about why the child is eating the food. Children like healthy foods and junk food, they just eat way too much food. Why? Because often due to broken families or other problems, the food becomes the best friend. Sometimes all these "food education" classes are totally missing the point. No teacher tries to find out why a particular kid is so overweight. Physical Education class for fat kids becomes a torture. These kids many times don't need exercise or a certain diet, but they need love and understanding and stability and normalcy. They need to know they are not alone.

Why is our nation obese? My theory is that mommy isn't home, says one Mom. She's at work. Who's watching what Latchkey little junior is eating and doing when he comes home from school? Nobody.

8. Parents can encourage kids to help with CHORES! They

can, for example, help in the yard and help clean the house. Instead of watching news that an American beat a Japanese in the Hotdog eating contest.

The crux of the obesity problem is that children eat when they're hungry. There are well known proportions of carbohydrates, (with a mix of high fiber and high density), protein and monosaturated fat that will keep adults and children from feeling hungry for four to six hours. All of this can taste good, and can be quickly (within about 20 minutes) prepared. Admittedly, the clean up time will be another twenty minutes which is twenty minutes longer than tossing into the trash a prepared food cardboard box.

Parents must set the example by eating healthy, take away the harmful from children, put in nutritious food, fed only at meals, and then get wide-spread community support for after-school and summer time physical activities that all children can participate in regardless of income level.

9. Its all about the parents. Its just another form of child abuse. We worry about second hand smoke, seat belts etc. Just make it a crime to treat your children as any other form of child abuse and hold the parents responsible. If the parents are fat most likely the kids are! Letting your child become obese is child abuse. There is NO EXCUSE for it. Poverty is not an excuse; prepared food is much more expensive than cooking at home. The government is not the solution and any of their "programs" are a waste of money, the lazy parents that are not parenting are the problem.

I am a CSA (Community Supported Agriculture) member at a farm, says one of the parents. As part of this membership I get the farm's fresh vegetables and fruits delivered to my door step every Tuesday. In addition to this, I also get to go to the farm and pick my own. This week I took my son blueberry & apricot picking. Last week we picked English peas and raspberries and the week before we picked strawberries. This gets him engaged and excited about eating what we have picked. It is also great exercise because it is very labor intensive to pick your own. Also, I live in a suburb of DC, so you too can do this even if you don't live in the middle of Iowa.

If you never introduce your kids to junk, they will not develop a taste for it.

As far as eating healthy, wash fruit and put it in a bowl in the middle of the fridge and/or on the counter where it's in plain sight and can be reached. See how quickly it will be gone. The bottom line is that most parents are lazy and ignorant and are abusing their children by cutting their lives short with poor diet.

10. Many articles are saying that there is now a rich/poor gap and the rich can eat better and exercise more. That's excuse. There's fruit, low fat dairy, frozen veggies at every store. Even peanut butter, if put on whole wheat bread can be healthy. And doesn't everyone have access to walking that costs nothing. Kids also love yoga. Show them some yoga moves in your home. Go to a garage sale and buy a workout video or something. Exercise even 2-3 times a week will make a difference. It's not a rich/poor thing. It's a lazy/not lazy thing.

11. Your children will eat healthy if you eat healthy. Don't short order cook for your children!!! If you are eating Baked chicken and broccoli for dinner, they should eat baked chicken and broccoli for dinner. Time and time again we see parents make macaroni and cheese for their toddler or preschooler if they don't like what's on the menu for dinner. A definite NO, NO!!! Give instead children fresh and/or frozen veggies since

birth and they will eat just about any vegetable that is placed in front of them. Don't stock up on junk food in the house. You can have treats after dinner once in a while (ice cream etc). All in moderation and it's only after a healthy meal has been eaten!! Snacks are usually healthy and NEVER prepackaged or processed!!! Learn how to read package labels!!! You would be surprised at the sodium, fat, and sugar contents in many prepackaged foods.

12. It is actually the disconnect between eyeballs and brain. Everyone's eyeballs and everyone's brain. "I was depressed" – yeah...but you weren't blind. "My parents were clueless" ....yeah but you weren't blind. "The food tasted so yummy" ... but you weren't blind. Look in a mirror. That's not a "normal" body. H-m-m......what's wrong with what my eyes are looking at. You're all a bunch of "It's not my fault" idiots who are too quick and too willing to blame someone else.

My kids have their mommy home 24/7 providing stability first and foremost. The icing on the cake, pardon the pun, is that they are also taught about healthy food and eating to live, not living to eat.

13. It's a combination of so many factors - the advertising, lack of low-cost entertainment options that include exercise that kids can do themselves, day care providers who get your kids started on junk food to save money (used mainly because the parents can't afford the cost of "good" daycare), and, despite the contrary views, good quality healthy food is expensive! It also requires more preparation time than prepackaged junk, and many of us are already stretched thin because we work all day, pick up kids from daycare, come home and cook, wash dishes, do laundry and try to have a little family time before we collapse and get up to do it all again tomorrow. Fresh

fruits and vegetables also don't last as long after they're purchased, so you have to make more trips to the grocery store.

14. Obesity is contagious — not like a virus is contagious, but in a social sense. If someone's friend becomes obese, that person's chances of becoming obese increase by more than half. Siblings and spouses also have an influence, although a reduced one — people whose siblings became obese were themselves 40 percent more likely to grow obese, while people whose spouses became obese were 37 percent more likely to.

15. Have children when you are in your 20s. That way you will have enough energy to keep up with the kids, do your job and maintain a household. Breast-feeding has many benefits for babies and also helps mother lose some weight.

We may conclude that overweight is no more a problem of adult and old generation, but kids and teenagers are not spared either. It is never too early to introduce youngsters to banish belly and lose weight information.

4

Potbellies More Dangerous than Just Overweight

Is your weight problematic? The answer is not as straightforward as you might think. Sure, there are scales and charts and different scientific methods of calculating "overweight and overall fatness," but determining your risk for heart disease may be more closely linked to *where* you carry your fat — not necessarily *how much* extra fat you're carrying.

When it comes to fat, "waist" is more important than "weight." Belly fat is a big predictor of health problems. Belly fat, for example, is the number one indicator that you are at risk for a heart attack. "Waist size should be one-half your height," says Dr. Mehmet Oz, a professor of surgery at Columbia University and director of the Cardiovascular Institute at New York Presbyterian Hospital; who now hosts a health-related TV show. For example, a 5'8" man should have a waist size no larger than 34 inches."

Dr. Oz and Dr. Roizen talk about five steps to losing this belly fat and living a healthier life.

1. Cut out all added simple sugars. Syrups and any foods that end in -ose (such as sucrose, glucose, fructose) should be removed from your diet.

2. Don't drink too much alcohol. "Alcohol increases the creation of triglycerides (you want that number under 100)," Dr. Oz says. "Plus alcohol is a simple carbohydrate."

3. Sleep. "When you don't sleep, the part of the brain that craves sleep has to make up for it," Dr. Oz says. " So it craves simple carbohydrates."

4. Manage stress. "Having a waist size more than half of your height is a great example of how you're coping with stress," Dr. Oz says. If your number is more than half, you run into progressive problems, and it also reflects that you're not coping with stress the way you want to.

5. Walk. If you walk at a good pace, you won't get hurt and you'll build up that core muscle that helps you get rid of the belly fat. Dr. Roizen says that walking also decreases insulin resistance. "Insulin is a mailman that takes sugar from your blood stream and puts it inside your cells," he says. "It decreases hunger because the hunger goes away when you get sugar inside the cells."

New research shows that adding several inches to the waist — even if body weight still falls within a normal range — markedly increases the risk of unhealthy plaque buildup in the arteries of the heart and the rest of the body. The research, conducted at the University of Texas Southwestern Medical Center in Dallas, appears in the August 21, 2007, issue of the Journal of the American College of Cardiology (JACC). According to the study, the relationship of the waist measurement to the hip measurement (known as waist-to-hip ratio) was much more closely tied to early, hidden signs of heart disease than other common measures of obesity, such as body mass index (BMI) and height/weight charts. In other words, get rid of that potbelly! And that's the primary aim of this book as you will find in the next Part II.

Learn to Measure Waist-to-hip Ratio (WHR) and Body Fat Percentage

Waist-to-hip Ratio (WHR):

To calculate your WHR, measure your waist circumference with a flexible tape measure. (If you have a visible waist, measure around the narrowest part of your abdomen.

Otherwise, take the measure at the level of your navel.) Record that number as your waist measurement. Then, measure around your hips — the widest part of your lower body, at or below the level of your pelvis. Record that number as your hip measurement. Now, take your waist measurement and divide by your hip measurement. That is your WHR. (For example, if your waist circumference is 30", and your hip measurement is 38": 30/38 = 0.79.) Higher WHRs indicate a greater proportion of weight carried as abdominal fat. If your measurements fall into the "at risk" category, start eating well and exercising to bring them down as soon as possible. Better still to follow like a religion what is tested and recommended in this guide.

Ideal waist-to-hip ratio :

For men, a ratio of .90 or less is considered to be safe.

For women, a ratio of .80 or less is considered to be safe.

For both men and women, a waist-to-hip ratio of higher than 1.0 is considered "at risk" or in the danger zone for undesirable health consequences such as heart disease.

The scoop on some standard height-weight charts:
According to height-weight charts, people are considered overweight if they carry more weight than what is usually expected for someone their height. For example, a woman of 5'8" who weighs 155 pounds is at a healthy weight. However, 155 pounds puts a woman of 5'4" in the category of moderately overweight, and a woman of 5'0" in the category of severely overweight. Although height-weight charts are useful, these charts are not practical for overly muscular people (since muscle weighs more than fat, an overly muscular person will be inaccurately categorized as "overweight"). Also, these charts do not measure fat

distribution, therefore, you should also measure waist-to-hip ratio for a comprehensive evaluation.

Body mass index (BMI): Body mass index (BMI) was created in order to standardize the height-weight relationship to a simple numerical scale. By using this chart instead of the height-weight chart, doctors use one number to determine whether you fall into a healthy weight range.

The formula for calculating your body mass index is: BMI = (Weight in pounds ÷ (Height in inches square) x 703. (Or simply use a BMI chart — they're readily available).

$$BMI = 703 \times \frac{weight\ (\text{lb})}{height^2\ (\text{in}^2)}$$

$$BMI = \frac{weight\ (\text{kg})}{height^2 (\text{m}^2)}$$

Here's example of 5'9" tall man who weighs 157 lbs.

BMI = (157 ÷ (69 inches square) x 703 which is **23.2**

Body Mass Index categories

Below 18.5 Underweight
18.5–24.9 Normal
25.0–29.9 Overweight
30.0 and Above Obese

As with the height-weight measure, BMI is not perfect, but it's a quick, inexpensive indicator that can be easily calculated during any physical examination. BMI charts do not work for overly muscular people (i.e., a bodybuilder), because as mentioned above, muscle weighs more than fat and will falsely categorize muscular people as overweight … and BMI charts do not take into consideration where your fat is distributed. Once again, it would be smart to track BMI and also measure your waist-to-hip ratio.

Body fat percentage:

Our bodies are made up of lean mass (muscle, bones and connective tissue) … and body fat. A measurement of body fat percentage shows how much overall body fat you have. These measurements are specifically useful for people who weigh a lot due to muscle mass. This reading validates the pounds are coming from lean body mass — NOT fat. It's also a useful tool for athletes trying to gain muscle and lose fat … and a fun tracking tool for people losing weight (to ensure you're losing FAT as opposed to lean body mass). If you'd like to investigate your "overall body fat percentage," you can get tested at a local gym or find a body composition lab that provides underwater weighing (the gold standard). You can also invest in a home scale that calculates body fat percentage, such as "Health O Meter BFM 687." Again, it would be smart to track total body fat and also measure your waist-to-hip ratio.

Extra Weight Fat Belly Body Shape and Health Risk

Extra weight at your waist increases risk of heart attack, high blood pressure, stroke and diabetes-but extra weight centered on the hips and thighs may not. Therefore banish belly and weight loss should be the aim and go hand in hand for good health.

To check out your "body shape risk," measure your waist at its narrowest point, and your hips (over your buttocks) at their widest point (as suggested earlier). Divide the inches measured at your waist by those measured at your hips.

An increase in health risks are related to a ratio that's greater than 1.0 for men, and 0.8 for women.

Belly Fat, Cortisol and Stress Connection: Cortisol levels are very relevant to weight control. Even if you have a perfect diet, if your cortisol is not held in check, you are likely to get fat -- and you'll get the worst kind of fat, which is excess abdominal fat. This type of fat causes the spare tire or dreaded "apple-shaped" body that puts you at higher risk of heart disease and diabetes.

You can naturally even out your cortisol levels -- and thus glucose (blood sugar) levels, since the interaction between the two is what usually leads to fat accumulation.

Cortisol (often called stress hormone) is a hormone normally secreted by the adrenal glands to regulate carbohydrate metabolism and blood pressure. In the often-cited "fight or flight" response, when you perceive a threat -- whether it's an oncoming car or an argument with your partner -- your body shifts into high gear, pumping out extra stress hormones to help you withstand the attack. Cortisol boosts your energy level during such stressful periods... yet too much of this hormone keeps the appetite stimulated and glucose production revved up. Excess glucose gets converted into fat, which the body stores in the belly for easy access.

This isn't really a problem if stress is a rare occurrence -- you cope with the problem, life calms down and cortisol levels go back to normal. However when you live in a state of constant, chronic stress (you know, problems at the office, overdue bills, college tuition, aging parents... life as usual for a lot of us these days) your body produces a steady stream of cortisol, which can create excess belly fat.

What you can do to make belly fat go away is to add a third mantra to the classic "eat less, exercise more" weight-loss formula. To banish belly fat and return to an optimal weight, Dr. Andrew Rubman, director, Southbury Clinic for Traditional Medicines, Southbury, Connecticut, says it's also essential to reduce stress. Though that may be easier said than done, Dr. Rubman says consistent practice of the following strategies can help your spare tire melt.

Emphasize high-quality, low-glycemic carbohydrates in your diet. The glycemic index is a measure of how fast a carbohydrate raises your blood sugar. To keep blood sugar on an even keel, the majority of carbs you consume should be healthful, low-glycemic ones, such as most fresh veggies and fruits and not high-glycemic such as syrups and sugars.

Make sweets only an occasional treat. The goal, of course, is to cut back on high-glycemic carbs. These lead to fluctuating blood sugar levels, which cause food cravings. Avoid these by saying no to candy, cookies and soft drinks, as well as fast foods, processed foods, chips and white bread.

Monitor food combinations. When hunger strikes, quiet your appetite and boost your energy with a healthful protein/carb combo. For example, try nut butter and whole-wheat crackers... low-fat yogurt and granola... a fruit salad sprinkled with walnuts... or turkey breast, lettuce and tomato tucked into a pita. Protein/carb combinations tend to reduce the impact of high-glycemic index foods by slowing their absorption and thereby reducing the speed at which they're converted to glucose and then fat.

Exercise, exercise, exercise. Thirty minutes of moderate-intensity exercise three to five times a week can help people lose weight and ward off heart disease and diabetes -- it also keeps stress in check. Some of the favorites are biking, skiing (a cross-country ski machine works too) and brisk walking.

Practice effective stress management. A great diet and regular exercise can be unfairly sidetracked by the high levels of cortisol that accompany ongoing stress, so it, too, needs to be regulated. Relaxation techniques such as meditation, deep breathing, progressive muscle relaxation, yoga and Tai Chi really do bring results. (Most of them are described in *"Art of Stress-free Living"* by Dr. S.S. Dhillon). In addition take short breaks instead of pouring a cup of energy in the form of coffee or tea, head outdoors for a 10-minute walk in the fresh air and sunshine.

Finally, you can think of that spare tire as "excess baggage" you don't need to lug around. In addition to eating right and exercising regularly, anything you can do to reduce stress will lighten your load -- in every way. This quote from *"Art of Stress-free Living"* says it all: "Diet and exercise alone are like a two-legged stool. It's more stable with the third leg, stress management."

Why Potbellies are Dangerous!

There are more specific scientific findings behind it being dangerous than simple cortisol connection. A protein in blood points to rising amounts of a particularly lethal form of body fat around organs, scientists say.

As levels of retinol-binding protein 4 (RBP4) rises, so do levels of "inter-abdominal fat" linked to an increased risk for heart disease and type 2 diabetes, the researchers say.

"Increased inter-abdominal fat is known to be associated with cardiovascular risk," said study co-author Dr. Barbara B. Kahn, chief of the Division of Endocrinology, Diabetes and Metabolism at Beth Israel Deaconess Medical Center, in Boston.

Reporting in the July, 2007 issue of *Cell Metabolism*, her team noted that increased "deep belly" fat around organs has long been linked to an increased risk for insulin resistance and type 2 diabetes. "The regulation of this protein may tell us completely new information about what really causes type 2 diabetes," said Kahn, who is also a professor of medicine at Harvard Medical School.

In the study, the researchers found that the amount of RBP4 in the blood accurately reflected the amount of fat surrounding the abdominal organs. That means that "RBP4 might be able to be used as a marker to indicate cardiovascular risk," Kahn said.

She stressed that RBP4 is not a cause of obesity. However, increased levels appear be associated with this particular type of abdominal-fat obesity.

In the study, Kahn and colleagues looked at biopsy samples of abdominal fat from 196 people. They found that more RBP4 is made in visceral (deep belly) fat compared with the subcutaneous fat that lies just beneath the skin. In addition, blood levels of RBP4 are greater in people who are obese. These people have double or triple the amount of RBP4 compared with normal-weight people.

"The gene expression of RBP4 is increased more in visceral adipose [fat] tissue -- the adipose tissue surrounding the internal organs -- than it is in the subcutaneous adipose tissue," Kahn said. So, levels of RBP4 are higher in people who have a so-called "visceral pattern" of obesity compared with people that have a subcutaneous pattern of obesity, she said.

In earlier research, Kahn's team also found that the levels of RBP4 were elevated in people with insulin resistance, people who are obese, and people with type 2 diabetes. This was also the case in healthy people with a family history of diabetes.

According to Kahn, there's ongoing research into drugs that could lower RBP4 levels.

But there's another tried-and-true means of lowering RBP4, she added.

"Levels can also be regulated by physical exercise," Kahn said. In prior research, her team showed that "people who benefited from an exercise program lowered their levels of serum RBP4 when they got more insulin-sensitive," she said.

Kahn had also shown in earlier research that teens who went on a low-carbohydrate diet along with an exercise program lowered their RBP4 levels.

One expert thinks that lowering RBP4 levels might help treat heart disease and type 2 diabetes.

"This study suggests that RBP4 can be a good biomarker to quantify visceral adiposity, which is closely linked to metabolic syndrome," said Dr. Tae-Hwa Chun, from the Department of Internal Medicine, Metabolism, Endocrinology and Diabetes at the University of Michigan. "This article also supports the notion that all the fats are not equal in their functions."

In experiments with mice, RBP4 decreases insulin sensitivity of muscle and liver tissue, which is considered a precursor to diabetes, Chun said.

"It is still not clear whether RBP4 regulates insulin sensitivity by controlling retinoic acid metabolism or by directly acting on muscle or liver cells," Chun said. "The drug Fenretinide, which is shown to lower RBP4 levels, has been already used as a chemotherapeutic agent for cancer. The side effects of the drug, however, need to be carefully weighed against its possible benefit for metabolic diseases."

In another report published in the same issue of the journal, a research team led by Bruce Spiegelman of the Dana-Farber Cancer Institute in Boston identified a gene called *PRDM16* that regulates the production of so-called "brown fat" in mice. Brown fat is a type of fat that actually generates heat and counters obesity caused by overeating.

"Brown fat is present in mice and in human infants, where it keeps them warm by dissipating food energy as heat, instead of storing it as 'white' fat," Spiegelman said in a prepared statement. "Human adults don't have much brown fat, but there is some, and from a therapeutic perspective, the question is whether that pathway can be reactivated."

The researchers hope their discovery will lead to new ways of treating obesity in humans.

You don't need to worry about these scientific findings, if you can reduce the belly fat by following nutrition and exercise program or the easy to follow specific techniques in this book.

SOURCES: Barbara B. Kahn, M.D., chief, Division of Endocrinology, Diabetes and Metabolism, Beth Israel Deaconess Medical Center; Tae-Hwa Chun, M.D., Ph.D., Department of Internal Medicine, Metabolism, Endocrinology and Diabetes, University of Michigan, Ann Arbor; *Cell Metabolism*, July 13, 2007

5

Humor: God didn't Want us Fat!

In the beginning, God created the Heavens and the Earth and Populated the Earth with broccoli, cauliflower and spinach, green and yellow and red vegetables of all kinds, so Man and Woman would live long and healthy lives.

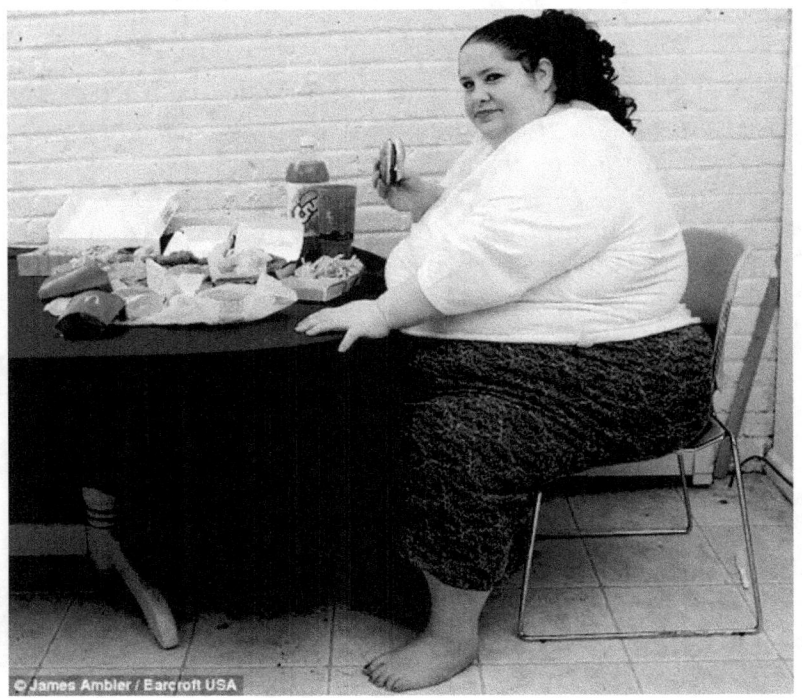

© James Ambler / Barcroft USA

Then using God's great gifts, Satan created Ben and Jerry's Ice Cream and Krispy Creame Donuts. And Satan said, "You want chocolate with that?" And Man said, "Yes!" and Woman said, " as long as you're at it, add some sprinkles." And they gained 10 pounds. And Satan smiled.

And God created the healthful yogurt that Woman might keep the figure that Man found so fair.

And Satan brought forth white flour from the wheat, and sugar from the cane and combined them. And Woman went from size 6 to size 14.

So God said, "Try my fresh green salad."

And Satan presented Thousand-Island Dressing, buttery croutons and garlic toast on the side. And Man and Woman unfastened their belts following the repast.

God then said, "I have sent you heart healthy vegetables and olive Oil in which to cook them."

And Satan brought forth deep fried fish and chicken, and juicy steak so big it needed its own platter. And Man gained more weight and his cholesterol went through the roof.

God then created a light, fluffy white cake, named it "Angel Food Cake," and said, "It is good."

Satan then created chocolate cake and named it "Devil's Food."

God then brought forth running shoes so that His children might lose those extra pounds.

And Satan gave cable TV with a remote control so Man would not have to toil changing the channels. And Man and Woman laughed and cried before the flickering blue light and gained pounds.

Then God brought forth the potato, naturally low in fat and Brimming with nutrition.

And Satan peeled off the healthful skin and sliced the Starchy center into chips and deep-fried them. And Man gained pounds.

God then gave lean meat so that Man might consume fewer calories and still satisfy his appetite.

And Satan created McDonald's and its 99-cent double cheeseburger. Then said, "You want fries with that?" And Man replied," Yes! And super size them!" And Satan said, "It is good." And Man went into cardiac arrest.

God sighed and created quadruple bypass surgery.

Then Satan created HMOs

If you don't share this and other information that keeps you healthy to five old friends right away there will be five fewer people laughing in the world.

PART II

6

The Solution

It's really amazing how simple things practiced regularly can place us in a mind-boggling 'healthy' level. In this simple technique using as little as five-minutes to as much as twenty-minutes a day we can reduce stomach which is essential to lose weight. If **"Banish Belly and Lose Weight"** using as little as "Five-Minutes a day" sounds unbelievable, it really is. But find yourself. This simple technique is not about diet, drug or vigorous exercise to risk your health. Will it work overnight? Almost 'Yes,' because you will start noticing the difference everyday starting with day-one. It will not only reduce your weight and stomach but will improve your overall health. It will eliminate digestive system problems such as gas problem, acidity, constipation, and cleanse your colon. It will help to keep prostrate healthy and fibroid of uterus under control. It will lower cholesterol, cure diabetes, and above all improve your physical and mental health.

With all the knowledge and experience and having written 12 guides related to health, I must admit that I have maintained proper weight within the weight chart. However, I could not reduce even 5 pounds naturally to keep in the lower range of the chart. My reason for lower range is not for appearance but a natural treatment for higher cholesterol level that I always had between 200 to 300. (By the way even 300 was not considered high in 1980s when I was writing my first book "Health, Happiness, and Longevity.") You will see later the actual data where cholesterol, triglycerides, HDL and LDL gets to a healthier level after few months practice of what you will learn here.

NOTE: This Part two is actual technique and next part three describes the science behind the technique and technicalities. The readers need to read part three primarily to understand the theory and to master the technique. We suggest you read this useful information carefully and find out yourself that why this technique is so effective.

7

My Personal Experience

My personal experience is what prompted me to write this guide. I am in my sixties and live in North Carolina on East Coast. I visit my son every 3 or 4 months who lives on West coast in Northern California - San Francisco Bay area. During each visit I gain between 4 to 8 pounds depending on the length of stay. Mostly because of my break from regular eating schedule and eating outside. Dark beer lunch with bay view. Enjoyment of vacationing comes along with enjoying various foods. So don't feel guilty folks if you enjoy vacation and food. It's part of happy living and does come with few extra pounds. During one of my visits from December 20, 06 to January 15, 07 my weight went to 166.2 pounds which was about 8 pounds more and this time during my visit between March 30 to April 10, 07, it was 162.8 pounds which was about 4 pounds more than my usual weight. During my last visit I brought down to my normal weight by increasing protein and decreasing carbohydrate in my diet. My exercise schedule was about the same.

It is during this April visit when I tested my new technique described in this guide. Although it was only 11 days visit but again I weighed about 4 pounds extra. I reached back in North Carolina middle of night, the next day as usual I weighed myself and it was 162.8 pounds. In the next 7 days I changed nothing in terms of diet or exercise but used this technique that I am giving in this book. My weight started to come down everyday (even when I was using my usual optimum diet and exercise) except one day that it went from 159.2 to 159.8 pounds. I usually don't drink by myself but happened to have two gatherings where I did took some alcohol. Moderate drinking is OK but not good during weight loss program. My weight on April 17, 07, almost exactly after one-week was 158 pounds. I don't know how much will be fat but my belt went down almost one-notch. I do understand that there will be some water loss. But I don't hesitate to call it a miracle technique for reducing belly and losing weight. The most effective among any method I have tested or written about weight loss.

8

Personal Stories of Overweight People!

Everyone has a story about overweight. Real stories. Real weight-gain. Real weight-loss. Real struggle. Real joy. Real diet discoveries from "Cave Woman Diet" to "Birdseed Diet." The real people who fight overweight everyday with every trick of the trade. Many of these good folks lose the battle at the end. Many succeed to keep weight off. From some we learn good tips. Some of these may sound like our own stories. Many of these find no easy solution that works. Hope we have one here that has worked. The stories are real but identity is withheld to protect privacy. Enjoy!!

Karen's Overweight Story: At my best, I have still been chubby. After having 2 children, I am stuck at 207 pounds. Sometimes I feel like it's not that bad- especially since obesity is common in my family. But other times, I look at myself in the mirror naked and am mortified. The thinnest I can ever remember being was probably somewhere around 140. I was anorexic and weak and got very ill. I went from being so obsessed about my body to being married and so secure and comfortable that I have gotten lazy. I don't feel motivated to diet and exercise at all- I think it's because I'm just so worn out from taking care of the kids and the house and so exercise is just another chore. I do want to look more attractive for my husband, but he is so accepting of me and loves me and thinks I'm beautiful no matter what- so there is really no real motivation there. I do want to be healthy and look good, but I'm so lazy! And I can't stop eating. I know my portions are ridiculous and I get my medicinal chocolate/ ice cream fixes far too often. I want to stop, but can't seem to commit to the change. I wish I could afford at least a gym membership-somewhere I could go to just get focused and not be distracted by everything in my house. I really think that I would have fun going to a gym and enjoy my time alone and that the pounds would just slowly melt off while I was focused on fun instead of just obsessing about my weight.

*****

Betty's Overweight Story: The following is Betty's weight story in her own words. Learn how she lost weight she had gained, the problems she encountered along her Weight Loss Journey, and how the experience changed her life...

Three years ago, life wasn't very much fun. I was weighing in at 175 pounds, which was a mite too steep for my 5'3" frame - even if allowing for the 'large bone/large frame' calculations.

My overall cholesterol was pushing 300; my legs ached continually from the extra weight; and it was a miracle I didn't have any 'wind' accidents.

I was 28 and still single, still working fast-food (internally & externally), still living at home, and still searching for that perfect diet. I tried every fad diet in the book and they all tasted like I was eating a book, so I'd fall back into my old habits and put my weight concerns on 'ignore'.

One night I was propped up in bed reading a wicked horror novel when I was seized with a pain in my chest. I ignored it, reaching for another chocolate covered cherry. It was Christmastime, and I loved those "Queen Anne" dark chocs. A couple of minutes passed, and I was again hit with pain, this time feeling as if I was being crushed by a steam roller - and not one by Fischer Price! This was genuine pain - more than heartburn and more than being frightened of the story I was reading.

To make a very, very long story short, I experienced a mild heart attack. At 28, I had no idea that I could be a victim of a heart attack! The ill effects of eating had caught up with me at this early age, even though heart problems were non-existent in my family history. All those cheese snacks, donuts, fried chicken, fried okra, fried cheese, pastries and heavy puddings had taken their toll.

When one faces a life/death experience, it's like getting hit in the face with cold water on a cold day. You wake up really fast!

Needless to say, my diet underwent a HUGE change. It was amazing to say the least! After all those years of unsuccessful dieting, I was losing weight this time. Why? Because I was committed to losing weight. I didn't cheat - I COULDN'T cheat! I knew the terrible consequences if I did. I learned that yes, you really can lose weight if you cut back on the quantity of food, and the types of food.

My weight loss took about 5 months and I've kept it off for about three years now. Though I've got my diet under control, I still need to keep motivated, because I know that if I allow it, my weight will return.

As for my personal life, I was married a year ago to a very wonderful man. I've graduated from fast-food to the medical field; I am studying to be a nutritionist. Perhaps I can pass along my experience to others and help them as others have helped me.

If you are struggling with your weight, I hope my story helps you to stay concentrated and to lose weight.

*****

Nancy's Overweight Story: I have always been overweight, since I was a kid. So when people say "I just wish I could get back to the size I was when I was in school or college, etc" I don't understand this. I have gained weight since college but when you start out overweight, it doesn't seem to make a huge difference. I have worked for a long time to really love myself and I have accepted my overweight body (for the most part, I think everyone has those "fat days" regardless of how thin/big they are). I have started trying to take better care of myself, instead of trying to "lose weight". I try to go for a walk at least 3-4 times a week and I have been cooking for myself which means more fruits and vegetables and good fats and not so much crap food! I am still overweight and I probably always will be but I am feeling so much better lately! So energetic!!

*****

Ida's Overweight Story: Being overweight has always been a huge problem for me. I was a chubby child and all through school I dealt with my weight issues. I hate it! People can be so mean against fat people. It is wrong! We are people too, we have feelings sometimes there is nothing to do about it. I played sports in school, lifted weights, ran, exercised all the dang time and guess what? I was still fat! I have tried diet pills along with exercise, still fat. I have been to a nutritionist...still fat. It is something that I have to deal with. The hardest part of it for me is my family. They make little comments like my mom sent me an outfit she bought. She said it's so big you should be able to wear it, it can wrap around me three times. I know she didn't mean to be mean but it still hurt my feelings. My mother-in-law telling me I can now go on a diet at my wedding reception, even though I had been dieting 6 months before the wedding! Luckily my husband loves me for me and loves me just the way I am. He likes "chubby" girls and says he wouldn't change me at all. He said he doesn't want me to loose weight, he just wants me to be happy. I am lucky that I have someone who is supportive even though he is skinny!

*****

John's Overweight Story: I broke my foot and so now I am in this gigantic cast which goes up to my knee. Since I got the cast put on about a month and a half ago, I've gained about 20 lbs I would say, though I haven't been able to step on a scale since they put it on (it's too big and heavy). I dread stepping on the scale after they remove the cast.

I'm not even going to estimate. I am over weight. I have been exercising with hand-weights and doing sit-ups, but that's about all I can do with my foot hurt and in a big cast. I can't wait when I can go out for a walk again. For a long time!

I need to lose about 50 lbs. Then I will be back to normal again....

*****

Helen's Overweight Story: I'm a twin, so I was only 4 pounds 13 ounces at birth. I weighed the "normal" amount for kids my age until I got into fourth grade. My parents divorced that year, and well, let's just say you can guess what happened next. Emotional eating. I was chubby from then on. I weighed 152 pounds at my high school graduation. Did I mention I'm 5 feet on a good day? And that the other girls in my graduating class weighed 100 pounds soaking wet?

When I went to college, things got worse. I was away from home for the first time, worried about events happening at home, and became a bit reclusive for a while. To comfort myself, I ate...and ate. Finally, after my sophomore year of college, I had a wake-up-call. Trust me, being the only 20 year old who doesn't wear jeans will do that for you. I saw a doctor, took the half of Phen-Fen that doesn't cause heart attacks, and lost a lot of weight really quickly. The problem was, I was nearly starving myself. I'd eat eggs for breakfast and dinner (or egg whites) and a piece of chicken with ½ can of green beans for lunch. If I ate more, I gained weight.

Eventually I went off the diet. Somehow, with exercise, I managed to keep the weight off for three years...three glorious years, where I wore tank tops (Did I mention I had a breast reduction at the age of 20? I went from a 42F to a 38B-imagine the freedom) for the first time in my life. I even wore a bikini. Then I got married and gained 15 pounds. Then I got pregnant and gained 60 more. Needless to say, it didn't all come off. I've tried over the years-I've tried hard. But eventually I've given up, after gaining a few pounds and throwing in the towel, declaring myself a failure again.

At this date, after birthing two beautiful children, I'm 48 pounds heavier than I was when I got married. And I want it off...and more. I don't want to be skin and bones. I don't even need to wear a single-digit size. But I do want to be able to walk into a restaurant with my kids and NOT wonder if I'm being judged if I (gasp!) order a milkshake.

So there's my story in a nutshell. I'm going to lose the weight this time. I have to. For me. For my kids. For my marriage. I'm happier when I'm at a healthy weight. I'm more self-confident, more likely to take adventures. It's time for me. Is it time for you?

*****

Kara's Overweight Story: I have always been heavier and I think I have a large frame. That doesn't bother me. It used to, but I've come to terms with the fact that there are some things I can't change and there are lots of people with bigger builds who aren't fat by any means.

These days I don't think I'd even want to be too petite/skinny. I just want to lose some excess weight and tone up a little. I'm bordering on being overweight for my height and build so I think I can afford to lose some.

I'm currently around 150 lbs. I want to get down to 140 lbs and see how I look. Ideally I'd love to drop a dress size or two.

*****

Beth's Weight Loss yo-yo Story: I would say I first started gaining weight when I was born (this is normal, right?). Seriously though, the trouble began long, long ago, in a galaxy far, far away when I was 17 and bought my first car.

Throughout all of my teenage years, I had to walk 2 miles each way to school and then BAM!, I suddenly cut 4 miles of daily walking out of my routine. Mind you, I was 110 pounds then and a teenager and could not be concerned with gaining a measly 5 pounds.

The trouble continued when, after graduation from a secretarial program at the technical college, I assumed my first desk job and stopped working at the roller-skating rink where I had spent about 3 nights per week on roller-skates. Hello, the next 5 pounds!

At the ripe old age of 21, I made the bold decision to move across the country and rent a house with my boyfriend and a roommate.

Can you say stress? It was also at about this point I figured I could eat the same portions as my boyfriend. What do you know? 5 more pounds. (Sneaky little buggers, aren't they?)

At 22, I moved back to my home town (yeah, the whole across the country thing didn't work out so well) and said hello to my first diet at all of 125 pounds. I did manage to lose

10 pounds that time by basically going vegetarian and cutting every bit of fat out that I could.

Well, I basically starved myself, but I was down to 115 again...for like a week! Nobody could uphold this diet, especially me, who could never, ever, go vegetarian.

We all know the old song and dance from here...back up to 125, down to 120, up to 130, down to 125, up to 135, up to 140! Over a span of eight years, I had yo-yoed myself to an all-time high of 142 pounds after Christmas 2001.

Of course, I was certain that the key was exercise and had tried the YMCA and Curves for a few years. I had great muscle...too bad you couldn't see it anymore!

Up and down, up and down, the scales went. I thought, "if I could only lose 10 pounds"...not willing to realize that I was, in fact, now 20 pounds overweight. You see, I have a unique disorder. Even though I knew the number on the scale was higher than it should be, and even though I was up to size 12 jeans, because my weight was distributed so evenly and I see myself every day, I didn't think I looked so bad...and then the holiday pictures rolled around. You know where I'm going here, don't you? You can't wait to get your pictures back from the developer because you know there are some really cute ones on that roll...and then you see yourself...and you say, what happened to my cute little figure?

So in January 30-years old, I started my longest and final diet. Mind you, when I started, I was only planning on dropping 10 pounds. I was a week or so into it and doing really well, when my motivation started to sag. I was having an especially hungry moment and I decided to surf the internet for some diet motivation. Where do you think I ended up? I saw some writings by this author, Dr. Dhillon who had used the best of Eastern traditions and Western Scientific knowledge!!!! I was so impressed by the simple but great information, that I spent the better part of two days reading all of the information and every bit I could get my hands on. Talk about gaining motivation! At that point, I decided this was it. I was going to lose every last bit of unwanted weight and keep it off. I started with wholesome Vegetarian diets that I thought will never try again; and ran with it from there. I don't necessarily count my calories, but I do try to create a balance of veggies, grains and meats at every meal, with minimal fat. I read labels religiously and many times decide the item isn't worth the amount of calories it contains. I also try to pay very close attention to when I am full and stop eating there. After a couple of minor miss-steps along the way, after 4½ months, I am 22 pounds lighter and at my goal weight of 120 pounds!

Imagine, I spent 8 years just hoping the weight would fall off by itself, without any work from me, and it didn't work. But it only took 4½ months after finally getting my butt and brain in gear and doing something about it! Something that I thought was futile and my biggest motivation now is the hope that I can stay in this happy place I am at.

*****

Sarah's Overweight Story: My name is Sarah and my official diet began on Valentines Day. My goal was to lose 50 pounds.

I have a job where I am on my feet all day long. I am a stylist. The only thing that looked good about me when I was so fat was my hair.

I had a quote that said: *"There is no wind beneath my wings because I'm too fat to fly."*

That is pretty sad now that I reflect on that.

I was too ashamed to give my weight stats. I started out at 205 pounds which was 50 pounds over for my height according to weight charts. It seemed like never ending nightmare. I was on a feeding frenzy....

I struggled with various diets to bring my weight back to 155 pounds so that is where I almost am!!!

I am 5'5" tall and have always carried my weight well. But when I look at old photos I cannot believe how fat I was. It is amazing what 50 pounds does!!!!

I may discover that I may need to lose a few more pounds, maybe to 135 or so. Another 15 pounds will not be easy to take off. I want this to be my last diet. And once I get there I NEVER want to gain this BITCH WEIGHT back again!!!!!!!

If you are reading this and thinking about going on a diet, I hope my story helps to encourage you. I will not lie. It has not been easy dieting. I was hungry at times but even when I was fat I was hungry ALL OF THE TIME!!!! So it was not that bad now that I think about that.

If you are dieting and read this please DO NOT GIVE UP!!! Miracles do happen!!!

I choose the photo at the beginning of my story to use because it made me think that I sorta like what I see in the mirror right now. I do not care if I am broomstick-thin.

The important thing is that I breathe easier now and standing up all day is not so hard anymore.

And I am in my normal weight range! And I have a yellow outfit that I can now fit into which I bought to help motivate me.

Right now, I am 2 pounds BELOW my goal weight! I have decided to lose just a FEW more pounds. This is what I am thinking. I want to never get over 150 pounds again. That means if I am at 145 or so that it will make it real easy to keep my weight in check.

*****

Zelda's Overweight Story: I was the lowest that I had ever been in life, totally depressed with myself for allowing my weight to climb to such heights, writes Zelda. I was now 50 pounds overweight and climbing up the scale with each passing day. No matter how hard I tried, I just didn't know how to stop the madness.

At age 35, it seemed much more difficult to shed the unwanted weight than it had been during my 20's. I wasn't quite as active now, as I had been then, either. And my cooking skills had excelled with time. My three layer fudge cake would put the corner deli to shame.

One day as I sat thinking, I pondered a lot about my younger days when I'd been thin. I remembered looking into a mirror whenever I got a chance to admire my sleek shape.

These days, I avoided mirrors at all cost. I used to wear bright colors and highly favored white. These days, I donned black. I used to wear tight fitting jeans and fancy skirts. These days, I wore vests and cloaks to hide my girth. It was at this point that I realized I had turned into a pudgy person who was beginning to sound a lot like Dracula. That thought was very scary.

I realized I had a problem. I was 50 pounds overweight. How could I lose the weight and keep it off? How could I stay on a diet and see it through?

I began to think about my younger thinner days again. I was so active back then; I loved biking, skating, jumping rope - all very basic, physical things. That evening, I bought a bike, a pair of skates, a jump rope and a couple of 2-pound weights. I even picked up a package of jacks to help bring out the kid in me. I made a pledge to myself that I would use my new and very inexpensive weight equipment at least four times a week, thirty minutes each time.

My diet menus would be a bit tougher. My family and friends were very fond of my gourmet cooking skills, and fortunately, none of them had a weight dilemma. So I promised myself that I would continue to bake but would limit my 'testing of the finished product' to one small serving or slice. I was also interested in seeking new ways to bake healthier treats and meals, so I made that part of my weight goals.

My daily diet consisted of a bowl of cold cereal for breakfast with 1 cup of fruit. I measured everything! I was so surprised to find that my usual 'helpings' were much too large. One cup isn't much more than a handful.

I cut out all daily snacks. Other than the skim milk that I put on my morning cereal, I enjoyed diet drinks for my beverage choice. I abstained totally from alcohol, which is very high in calories. I used 'fake' butter and 'fake' sugar, too.

Lunch consisted of one sandwich and one bowl of Campbell's soup (1 serving size) or a small lettuce and tomato salad with 1 Tablespoon of dressing on the side. Generally, my sandwich was made with 1 slice of lean deli meat, lettuce, tomato and a bit of mustard. I was never a mustard lover, but if I could drop 50 pounds, I'd gladly give up my Mayo.

Although pickles are very low in calories, I opted against them due to the high sodium content. I was also very aware of the sodium content in the deli meat and made my selections very carefully.

When I tired of deli meat, I roasted a bit of chicken and sliced it into thin slices for my sandwich. I opted not to eat red meat during my diet.

Dinners were my most difficult diet dilemma. I would come home from work, very tired, and I longed to just chill out in front of the television with my traditional bag of hot buttered popcorn. I missed those comforting times a lot! I kept my dinners to one slice of meat, 2 cups of steamed vegetables, one slice of bread and one box of sugar-free gelatin for dessert. Sometimes, I think it was the only thing that kept me going - that one box of gelatin at the end of the day! It may seem like a lot, but it's only 40 calories for the entire box and it's really filling.

I lost about 12-15 pounds a month when I was dieting. I hit three weight loss plateaus: one after I had lost 15 pounds, another after I had lost 32 pounds, and another when I had lost 41 pounds. I seemed to stay at the same weight for a week or more during these plateaus. It was very depressing, and I felt like giving up many times. But I stayed the course and when almost 4 months had passed - I WAS AT MY WEIGHT GOAL!!! But I was not sure about keeping it up!!!

I celebrated by riding my bike through the woods of a local state park on a bright, sunshine Saturday morning. I cannot express the joy that I felt over my personal success. The sun was on my face, and the wind was blowing through my uncombed hair and I felt like the most lucky creature on God's green earth! I felt beautiful inside like never before.

*****

Tina's Teenage Goblin Overweight Story: On October 31st, I'll celebrate my 30th Birthday. Birthday's are a bit different for those of us born on celebrated holidays. Our lives and personalities tend to take on some of the attributes of the holiday. In my case, I became a Goblin during my teenage years, meaning that I liked to gobble up everything in sight.

I felt fat, powerless, stressed out, and just flat ugly.

There were so many issues to deal with during that uncertain phase - skin problems, makeup decisions, that first car, and of course - getting a boyfriend. I discovered that the more I tried to adjust and achieve all my hopes and dreams, the deeper I sank into the bowels of the gourmet feeding pond.

Everywhere I turned; there was some form of unhealthy food tempting me. At school, it was the fried foods - French fries, fried steak, and fried chicken. There was always the option of bringing my lunch, but unfortunately, my mom supported the theory that a healthy lunch consisted of peanut butter and jelly sandwiches, a bag of name-brand potato chips, and a packaged cupcake - usually of the snowball variety. Mom loved the color pink.

During recreational times, I was again hit with unhealthy choices. At the movies, there was the luscious hot buttered popcorn. At the zoo, there was the cotton candy. At the football games at High School, there were chili dogs and nachos. And at home, there were those pink snowballs that mom loved so much.

What I considered as recreation, certainly was not! When I wasn't sitting at the movies, I was sitting at a football game, and when I wasn't sitting at a football game, I was sitting at home watching television, or talking on the phone to my very small circle of friends.

By the time I reached 17 my weight had soared to 215 pounds. What made that so bad was the fact that I was 5 feet tall. Can you imagine how embarrassed I was? How fat I felt? How unattractive I felt? Truth is, I felt terrible, and thought of death continually. I was always worrying about dying. Why? I felt that I was so large, that my health must certainly be at risk.

At least, according to the dentist, it was. One night I awoke with a terrible toothache and the following morning, mom took me to the dentist. He told mom that I needed to lose weight, and then sent me home. He attributed my pain to an overdose of sweets, even though several weeks later another dentist discovered a cavity. I suppose if I had accidentally cut off my finger, he would have said the same.

So to recap, I was fat, young, miserable, and one tormented soul.

And now, I suppose you are anxious to learn how quickly and how successfully that I lost weight. You may be surprised. You may not be. This is my story...

It was January 1st, the beginning of a new year. I was 19 and I had really enjoyed the feasting of the holidays. I was disgusted with my overweight self, but I didn't want to do the diet thing ever again. Each time I went on a diet, I ended up weighing more than when I had started the diet. So, what to do? I wasn't sure, but I did know that I didn't want to go through life at that size. I was tired of being fat.

On January 15th, I had made the decision of a lifetime. I wasn't going on a 'diet' per say. I had chosen to simplify my life. I decided that I had worried long enough over my weight. From this point out, I was going to keep my life simple. I was going to make a set of rules and follow them, and I wasn't going to worry anymore about the extra unwanted weight. If my plan worked, then great. If not, I would know that I had done everything humanly possible to lose the weight. I also knew that I would at least be healthier, if not thinner. And I was determined to be happy - fat or thin!

My simple plan! I promised myself that I would only make healthy food choices. I decided that I would cut out all snacks and eat three meals a day. I promised myself that I would have one 'normal-sized' plate or one bowl for each meal of the day. And if I missed a meal, then it was gone forever. No double-meal for me.

I decided that I would walk one mile every day, rain or shine, health permitting. I made a promise to myself that I was going to stick with this plan until January 1st of the following year.

I made a promise to myself that I would only weigh once a month, on the 1st of every month. If I wasn't losing weight, I didn't want to become depressed about that. If I was, then great. This was going to be done as simply as possible. I had other things in life that were out there, waiting for me. I was going to forget all of this dieting 'crap' and get on with life. I was sick and tired of worrying about my weight, tired of being depressed over my weight.

Choosing to simplify my food intake choices was my way of solving my overweight problem and sweeping it aside so I could concentrate on these other things - wonderful, good things in life that until now I hadn't felt that I deserved. All of this, simply because I was overweight. It was really quite nuts.

Well, enough was enough! I made a promise that I wasn't going to worry about being overweight anymore! I would follow my simple plan, choose healthy foods, and be true to myself. What happened would happen. I would accept that - whether I was met with defeat or with success and I would continue to live my life without being filled of constant thoughts of being overweight. Of being - as my dentist had phrased - obese, a word that I really do not like.

It wasn't easy passing up cake and ice cream for apples and oranges. It wasn't easy passing up fried chicken for baked fish. It wasn't easy passing up broccoli piled with creamy cheese sauce for plain steamed broccoli. And those three meals a day seemed very sparse at times. I was tempted so many times to toss a bag of the extra-butter variety popcorn into the microwave and enjoy it with a glass of REAL soda.

But I was true to myself and I stayed the course.

It wasn't easy some days, walking that meager one mile. When it rained, I went to the mall to walk. When it snowed so badly that I was unable to go outside, I walked the mile inside the house. It wasn't easy, but I was true to myself and I stayed the course.

My results?

The following year on January 1st, my weight had dropped 102 pounds. My wardrobe from the previous year had been donated to charity. Even then, I could hardly believe that those simple changes had made such a huge difference in my weight - in my very life. I went from a size 22 to a size 4. Imagine that!

Am I happier? Sure. And I feel terrific. My sick days were also cut by at least 3/4. I used to suffer from continuous heartburn. Not anymore. I used to have bouts of nausea. Not anymore. I used to have trouble breathing some days. Not anymore. I used to snore very loudly at night. Not anymore.

If you are trying to lose weight, I would encourage you to try to simplify your diet. Cut out all of the items that aren't of the basic nature of life. Don't allow anyone else to influence your decision to lose weight. Stay the course and be true to yourself, because yes, you are worth it! Sometimes, friends mean well, but they can do more harm than good.

I am always in search of diet recipes to spice up my life and to keep me motivated. Keeping the weight off after my diet is an everyday battle. Yes, I have treats every now and then, but I know that if I don't work hard and watch what I eat, and exercise, I'll gain it all back, and probably more. I don't want to ever have to lose weight again.

*****

William's Overweight Story: I hope that my story helps anyone struggling with the very stressful task of losing weight.

I live in Texas; I have all my life. Everything is big here – the state, the tall tales, and especially the amounts of food available. Due to the tropical-like climate there's a party going on somewhere all year long. Generally, people here like to grill a lot. They like tailgate parties at the beach. They love chili recipes. Beef is big, and they really like beef. Seven years ago, I liked it all.

I was thirty-five and had no health problems whatsoever, thank God! However, I didn't like what I saw when I looked into the mirror each day. I didn't like shopping for clothes. I especially didn't like attending pool parties. I felt like '*Free Willy*' at those types of events. In fact, I was even called that a few times because it related to my name, as well as my size back then.

One day, my emotions started caving in on me. I wanted to lose weight. I didn't want to be that huge all my life. I was single and had never been very successful in getting dates.

In fact, that's what prompted my weight loss voyage. I had asked a lady (let's call her Cindy) to accompany me on a date to a movie. Cindy was a very pretty lady, and had been quite friendly towards me during the three months I had known her. We got along fabulously and shared the same sense of humor. However, I'll never forget her cruel response that evening. "Are you kidding, Will? We'd have to call 911 to have them extract you from the theater seats once the flick is done. No way!"

I laughed. It was painful. Somehow I managed to get through the next ten minutes, then I cried my eyes out on the drive

home. It was a long drive, too, and a miracle that I could see the road through my wall of tears.

I loved food – all food. I had read miraculous stories about people who had lost massive amounts of weight through the Cabbage Soup Diet. For the next month I survived on cabbage. I ate cabbage soup. I stir-fried shredded cabbage using nonfat cooking spray. I made cabbage coleslaw using nonfat Mayo. I ate boiled cabbage, steamed cabbage, raw cabbage, even grilled cabbage (it was that grilling instinct that surfaced unexpectedly).

During this transition, I had made a pack with myself that I wouldn't weigh until a month had passed. The faithful day had arrived, and when I stepped on the scales I was shocked to note the 41-pound weight loss! My clothes had become extremely loose and I had even had to poke a new hole in my belt so that it could be buckled. However, I was totally amazed about the huge drop.

My goal was to lose 126 pounds. I only had 85 more to go! Another thing that I kept in the back of my mind is the fact that just about everyone needs or wants to lose 25 pounds. (Even thin people.) So if I could make it down another 60 pounds, I'd be in sweet heaven.

During the following week, I began to have some dizzy spells so I contacted my doctor. Once I met with him, I explained my 'diet plan' to him. When he began lecturing me on the dangers of how I had went about losing weight, I sat up and took notice.

He had me meet with a nurse who specialized in nutrition. She counseled me on the correct way to go about losing the weight that I needed to lose. Also, the doctor gave me a prescription for *Merida*, a diet medication that helped curb my appetite.

I was concerned that once I winged myself off the cabbage plan that my weight would return. It didn't! Three and a half months later, I had dropped another fifty pounds. From there it got much easier because I could see the end results! I could visualize a window in the near future! I was slowly escaping from '*Fat Hell*'.

Needless to say, I met my goals and have worked hard in maintaining my weight over the years. Sometimes, I still long to binge. I don't think that will ever go away. However, I like my new self more than I want to binge. I eat smart, I visit the gym two times a week, and I don't mind going to those pool parties so much anymore! Hey, thanks Cindy!

*****

Jack's Overweight Story: I would like to relate my experience of being fat.

As a retired Marine I have been burned and blasted but nothing can compare to how I felt this past winter when my weight shot up from about 150 to 192.

I am 64 and my eating and drinking routine were normal routine. I was totally embarrassed and humiliated. My clothes wouldn't fit and I was ashamed to be seen in public. Other than an occasional glass of water and handfuls of peanuts I gave up eating and drinking and lost 32 pounds in less than 3 weeks.

It was not an easy transition. My stomach, legs and feet were swollen and I itched horribly. Down to 160 my lower stomach began to ache, a good night's sleep was impossible.

I now weigh 150 and I feel a great deal better. My stomach still hurts and I don't have much of an appetite. Usually I will have kielbasa (sausage) and eggs for breakfast, maybe some cookies and milk or a peanut butter jelly sandwich during the day.

I am not going to be fat again. I would not recommend this method of loosing weight. Looking back I probably would have been better off going on rice and raisins. Years ago before Viet Nam we were given a sock full of rice and raisins and told to get going, live on the sock for a week and you better not get caught. I didn't get caught, nor did my weight go up or down.

My attitude about fat people has changed. I used to think that fat people were simply piggish and ate too much. Now I am not so sure. Admittedly I am not as physically active as I was but for the sudden weight gain to happen is beyond me.

One of my old Marine pals has a daughter that was very fat. At Christmas when I visited she had lost nearly 150 pounds, I didn't recognize her when she answered the door. She was absolutely gorgeous! Later this summer at a picnic I saw her and she was again fat, wearing a mu-mu. It must be devastating because at 192 I hated myself in the mirror every morning when I shaved. I have no idea what the answer is.

After I started eating again I was buying all this diet, fat free crap that tasted like crap and was more expensive than real food. I ended up throwing it out. I now eat only when I am absolutely hungry. Main fare is kielbasa (sausage), fried eggs or an omelet, micro waved potato and toasted rye bread with dairy butter on the bread and potatoes, salt and pepper, banana and a glass of regular milk.

*****

Shelly's Overweight Story: I desperately needed to lose 100 pounds. In fact, for most of my life I had needed to lose 100 pounds. I had been an overweight child and the weight had carried over into adulthood. How one day at an amusement park changed my life forever.

It was a blistering hot day at the amusement park. The concrete added to the heat of the Texas August sun. At least the kids were happy, I thought as I watched them wait to ride the mini-roller coaster. I had left for a few moments to purchase a couple of ice creams for them to munch on as they waited in line, thinking that the coolness would help abate the heat. Funny, but the kids didn't seem as hot as I was. Then again, they weren't overweight either.

I had been grossly overweight as a child. Kids had been cruel, placing everything from balloons to marshmallows in my desk seat when I had attended school. I was so glad that my own kids had maintained normal weight.

Finally, they reached the front of the line to board the roller coaster. I was going to wait on the sidelines while the kids enjoyed the ride. They were boarding now and as I went to leave, the man in charge of loading everyone on the ride stopped me.

He told me, "You're too heavy to ride. You'll have to wait over there." He glanced meaningfully at the unfinished ice cream cone, his face clearly indicating why he believed I was too heavy. Or at least, that's how I interpreted things.

I felt as though I had been doused with a bucket of ice water - even amid all the searing heat around me! "I hadn't planned on riding," I managed to tell the man. It was a kid's ride, for goodness sake! And where was a trashcan so I could chunk the idiotic cone?

The man just stared at me, then delivered a disgusting glance to the cone, and then he just walked away. I felt confused, hurt, and a bit lost. And embarrassed. The place was jammed and the small confrontation had created a scene. More than a few people stood in line whispering behind their hands.

I was so bothered by the incident that I couldn't sleep that night. The next morning I made a decision to lose weight - all the excess weight. I was tired of feeling like I had a dead Albatross tied around my neck. Yes, I had been on tons of diets in the past, but this time I knew I was going to be successful!

I made an appointment with a physician who was very eager regarding my decision to lose weight. He suggested some basic tests that came back with some startling results. I had a thyroid problem. I also knew that my weight was in part due to poor eating habits but the thyroid was also a significant contributor.

It didn't happen overnight. At times it was very tough to resist temptation, but I stuck with my decision and was true to myself. A year and a half later, I was 100 pounds thinner!

Many times, I have thought back to the incident in the amusement park on that hot summer day. Sometimes, it just takes a huge mental shake to get a person seriously thinking about what they need to do.

*****

Coty's Cave Woman Diet Story: In spite of its name, this diet does not include being dragged by the hair, hunting with clubs or skinning big game. Though you might feel good enough to do all of those things. What it does include is a return to our evolutionary roots.

As a student of anthropology, I read every book I can find on ancient hominids and their culture. In January, while cruising Amazon for something new about our primitive cousins, I came across two books on ancient hominid diets. Out of curiosity, I ordered them.

In a nutshell, about 12,000 years ago the last Ice Age ended. Within 2,000 years of the ice sheet receding, agriculture began and new foods became the staple they are in today's diet. This new diet, called Neolithic, had an immediate effect on human health. Skeletons of Neolithic farmers show poor nutrition compared to the previous generations of hunter-gatherers. They died younger, were shorter, had more cavities in their fewer teeth and showed the first evidence of obesity.

The problem with the new diet of the Neolithic period was that we didn't evolve to eat those new foods. The small human digestive tract is unique among primates. We have only one stomach and a relatively short large intestine. We are more suited to digesting and extracting nutrients from meat, fruit, nuts, and some vegetables.

This was of particular interest to me since I knew I was allergic to wheat and was also lactose intolerant. If I couldn't digest those items, maybe there were other items I couldn't digest and just didn't know it.

After reading both books, doing some research on the Internet and at my local library, I fashioned a diet for myself. And the Cave Woman Diet was born.

On January 16 following year, when the last kid returned to college, I began my diet. Since the previous January, I had been exercising, lifting weights and generally killing myself to lose a grand total of ten pounds. And it took a year! Not a very satisfying result from so much effort.

I began by purging the kitchen of every slice of bread, every cracker, every package of pasta, and every cream-filled pastry. I was ruthless.

Next, I went to the store and bought meat. Beef, pork and chicken. Also, fish and shrimp. Then I hit the produce section. Fresh vegetables and fruits nestled in the shopping cart next to nuts and dried fruit (without sugar added) and eggs. The rules for eating were simple. Eat nothing that couldn't be found in nature. Eat only when I was hungry, even if it was every two hours. And eat only enough to satisfy my hunger. No gorging.

I began my eating day at 9 am. I scrambled an egg in a small amount of butter and topped it with a dash of cheese. At 11 am, I was back in the kitchen eating pastrami or corned beef (not processed, but from the deli). Just a couple of slices rolled inside a thin slice of cheese.

At 1 pm, I had lunch. Usually a left over item from dinner the night before. Pork chops, a stuffed pepper, a ground beef patty. Whatever. I made a small salad to accompany this with a teaspoon of salad dressing.

Between three and four in the afternoon, I was hungry again. This is when I got out the fresh fruit and nuts. Usually apples and walnuts. I munched them while I fixed a dinner of steak, chicken, pork or fish. I also prepared the fresh vegetables for the meal. I'm partial to broccoli, cauliflower and carrots, but I also ate snow peas, mushrooms and other vegetables, though no corn.

By eight or nine that night it was time to drag out the fruit again for something to snack on.

At the end of 5 days, I had lost three pounds and my chronic indigestion. Goodbye Tums! And I was never hungry since I ate all the time. Previous dietary study indicated that to change our metabolism it is necessary to eat often. This reprograms the body to stop storing fat.

The second week I dropped four pounds and my energy level skyrocketed. I was not just cleaning house, I was cleaning closets and kitchen cabinets and organizing items for a yard sale. Interestingly, I had no more sinus headaches or joint pain and had eliminated over the counter decongestants and arthritis pain relievers.

At the end of six weeks, I had lost twenty pounds, my clothes no longer fit and I had energy to spare. I was sleeping better and my anxiety level was greatly reduced. I felt better than I had in years.

I had continued a modified version of my daily workout during this diet period. Chronic back pain plagued me since my twenties and I used exercise to keep my muscles from seizing up. I had to wonder if my diet would have been as successful without the twenty minute a day workout. So, at the end of my third week, I put my wheelchair confined husband on the diet. He lost 12 lbs! A man who cannot move lost weight.

I was definitely onto something here.

I thought at the end of six weeks, it was safe to add a few goodies back into my diet. I missed a few things like a slice of bread with my meat and cheese and an occasional sip from a root beer float. Only in moderation, of course.

Big Mistake!

Those small indulgences made me sick. Tummy ache, diarrhea, headache. It didn't take a rocket scientist to figure out that modern foods were making me sick and probably had been all my life. That was pretty strong motivation to continue the Cave Woman Diet.

I am now at my ideal weight. I no longer suffer with indigestion and allergies. And I am more energetic and productive than ever. My coaching business is taking off. My writing business is flourishing. And I feel and look better than I have in years.

So, get out your loincloth, sharpen your stone tools and become a Cave Woman! Eat the way Mother Nature designed us to eat. Once you break the addiction to grains and sugars, you will never want to touch them again.

Common questions people asked about "Cave Woman Diet."

Why do we need to eat every 2-3 hours? The reason we have to eat every 2-3 hours is to convince our bodies there is no longer a need to store fat. You see, fat is our body's natural fuel. We substitute sugar and grains for fat and then we eat only 2-3 times a day. Our body is saying, "Hey, we better save up on fuel. There's not much coming down the pipe. Let's hold onto this extra fuel." By eating small amounts of food every 2-3 hours, we are telling our body that times are good. There is no famine on the horizon. We can have all the food we want anytime we want it. This is what changes our metabolism. Once our body gets the message, which can take 2-3 weeks, then it starts throwing away all that fat it stored in preparation for hard times. As long as you eat the right things, in smaller portions, you'll be fine.

Why did our ancestors start eating cereal grains in the first place? Ah, progress and civilization. But, actually, overpopulation is the real answer to this question. Hunter/gatherer societies of the Paleolithic period could travel hundreds of miles if necessary to follow constantly migrating game. But about 10,000 years ago that became nearly impossible. Everywhere they traveled, they ran into other people doing the same thing. And being cursed with a big brain they decided to settle down in small societies, domesticate animals for their consumption and grow their own vegetables and fruits.

Sounds like a great idea, but they had to improve on it. Without refrigeration and canning and with only rudimentary ideas about curing meat, they decided to grow something they

could store more easily. Potatoes were easy to grow and kept forever in a cool, dark place (like a cave). Grains could be turned into other food products and kept for long periods of time. These new products were also more filling and fed more people. It made perfect sense at the time for primitive people. It makes no sense now.

Why not exercise! It's good for you? Yes, it is. No one advocates giving up exercise. The point is, it is not necessary to work out vigorously to lose weight. Not if you follow the Cave Woman Diet. Did you know that our ancestors only worked 2-3 hours a day? Yep, that's right. They weren't lazy, it just didn't take much time to meet their basic needs. The men usually hunted game, either big or small, and the women gathered wild fruits and vegetables. Then they sat around eating or drawing on the walls for the rest of the day . Modern humans work 12-14 hours a day, work out to the point of exhaustion or injury and yet are fat and suffer disease. Doesn't it make you wonder what the ancients were doing right?

I've tried to give up sweets but I can't, I crave them? This is called the joys of addiction. Did you ever get irritated with a smoker? Well, welcome to the club. It doesn't matter what you are addicted to, cigarettes or sweets, it's still an addiction and it's just as hard to kick. But just as surely as cigarettes threaten your health, the wrong foods threaten it, too. I know this sound like a broken record, but if you are using sugar or carbohydrates for fuel, then your body is still storing fat. Make your body burn the fat for fuel like it was designed to do. It may not be easy, but then if it were, there would be no smokers and there would be no obese people.

Why the government advocate food pyramid? This is a great question with a complex answer. First it seemed simple. Corporate greed! Government conspiracy! Medical cover-up!

But that's only part of the story.

Food production is an economic commodity and a powerful tool in controlling the masses. Early state societies used it for that purpose. Ye Old History Book will confirm that the feudal lords obtained their high place in society and their wealth from food production. It has become a way of life in our culture and it isn't going to change anytime soon. Not unless we change it.

The whole modern concept of nutrition is actually a product of 20th Century technology. When scientists first began to identify vitamins and nutrients, they built the food pyramid on their findings. They had to find foods that contained these vitamins and nutrients. With typical cultural bias, they looked at foods we were all ready eating - modern foods - the wrong foods.

So, darn it, it wasn't a conspiracy.

However, we now know that it doesn't work. We can get vitamins and other nutrients by eating the right foods for our bodies. We can conquer stored fat by changing our metabolism. We can stamp out diabetes and autoimmune disorders by returning to our roots. We can do it all with a cultural food change.

*****

Larry's Birdseed Diet Story: It was diet #666, I am almost sure of that. Nonetheless, I was determined to succeed because I was sick and tired of the weight, sick and tired of sounding like a wheezing tea kettle whenever I had to climb steps.

Yes, I was on a diet. Yes, I was determined. But it was the birdseed that opened my eyes to success! My total weight loss on this diet was 34 pounds and I have maintained my current weight for over three months.

It began last fall. I am fortunate to reside in the beautiful state of Arkansas where the trees turn into living masterpieces during this colorful time of year. This time, I intended to enjoy those luscious colors and relax in the Ozark Mountains by using my well-earned 3 week vacation.

I also had another goal in mind, that being to lose a blasted 30 plus pounds that had leaded me down. The holidays were just around the corner, and I knew that if I didn't chisel off the unwanted (and un-needed) weight, then I would only add to it over the holidays.

To accomplish my weight loss, I decided to leave the cupboards empty in my rented cabin. Going out to eat would take time and thought, and was just the thing I needed to help me stick to my diet plan.

The first week just flew by. I must admit that I was a bit sore from not being used to climbing and hiking the woods. In the evenings, I would come back to my cabin and just fall into bed. I slept like a log every night until the sun hit my face the next morning.

The second week I was feeling a bit lonely and wished I had brought along my dog, Lance, for company rather than leaving him in the care of my apartment roommate. I spent those evening hours reading, relaxing and listening to the small radio that I had brought along for company, thought it wasn't quite Lance.

At the beginning of the third week, I was thrilled to discover that my clothes were loose! I had also dropped 2 belt notches, so my plan was working! I had faithfully kept to my diet when eating, choosing healthy foods such as fresh bread, lean meat - mostly fish, steamed veggies, and fruit for dessert. I was also making a point to drink more water and my skin looked healthier for it, or perhaps it was that fresh mountain air. Nonetheless, I felt like a million bucks. My dog Lance probably wouldn't even recognize me when I returned home; I thought one morning to myself.

It was my last night at the cabin. I regretted having to leave for home the next day and be faced with once again returning to work rather than being able to play in the mountains. It was a lot more fun!

I couldn't sleep that evening because I was so anxious from everything circling in my head. And I was so hungry. It was the first time that I felt famished since I had begun my diet.

I tossed. I turned. The moon was so bright that night and it was rather chilly. I was so hungry at this point I felt like going out into the mountains and finding a bear to cook! I was desperate. All the stores in the tiny nearby town had closed their doors hours ago.

Then I remembered a small convenience store that I had visited one morning for a pack of gum. It had reeked of fish, but I was desperate so I got dressed and made the ten-mile drive into town.

I was shocked. CLOSED stood posted on the front door of the stinking little store. Now what?

Despondent, I returned to my cabin. My stomach was doubled from the hunger. I undressed and climbed into bed, but I couldn't sleep because of the hunger.

Then I remember the birdseed!

I had brought along some birdseed to feed the birds so I could watch them from my cabin window each morning. I could eat the birdseed!

I raced to the sealed pail, popped off the top and began shoveling the birdseed into my mouth as fast as I could. I also choked once, and it's not a food I would recommend for taste.

After a minute or two, I stopped when I saw myself in the full-length mirror visible from my bedroom. I looked incredibly stupid, my mouth pasted with stray seeds. I felt like a giant dodo bird.

I laughed at myself, first whimsically, then louder, and finally I laughed so hard that I almost lost my breath. My Birdseed Diet, I thought. Is this what it had come down to? I was a pitiful, although funny site to behold.

But seeing myself in this frantic state made me realize that I had the power to control what went into my mouth. I had chosen the birdseed. I had prepared my cabin to have nothing edible in it for those 3 weeks. I thought that I had covered all my bases. And now, I realized that I would always be faced with food choices. That birdseed didn't walk into my mouth. I put it there, desperately put it there.

I suddenly realized from that moment on I would have to begin facing these food choices and learn when to say yes, and when to say no.

I went on to lose a total of 34 pounds. I have only kept off my weight for about three months, but I know that this will be a lifelong endeavor.

And now you know about my Birdseed Diet. I hope my story inspires you! Good luck to all!

*****

Harold's Diet Story: Twelve pounds in ten days during my 10-day Hawaiian vacation, feasting on pineapple Mai Tais, succulent pit-roasted piglet, and coconut rum cakes... But it was my vacation. Sad but so, the party is over and it's time to float back down to Mother Earth. I was floating down a bit heavier than before my vacation, but I was serious about getting the excess off.

I gained 12 pounds in 10 days, so I should be able to lose 12 pounds in 10 days, right? When succulent pit-roasted pigs fly.

Why?

I ate approximately 42,000 calories OVER my daily calorie requirement in order to gain those 12 rotten pounds of Hawaiian flab. I will need to expend that many calories in order to lose those 12 pounds.

As a note, we are assuming that these pounds are 'fat-stored pounds' rather than 'water-stored pounds'. In simple terms, I actually ate those 42,000 calories - not just sodium-laden foods that generally confuse the old scale.

My normal weight is 150 pounds. If I walk 3 ½ miles per hour, I'll burn about 180 calories for a 2-mile walk. If I run, I'll only burn about 20 calories more.

Even if I walked for 8 solid hours, I'd burn less than 1 pound. If I also decreased my daily calorie requirement by 500 calories, I'd lose about 1 pound for the week.

So, as we can see - it takes a lot of effort to work off excess weight. Yet, it was so easy to gain. Why?

Mixed drinks are extremely high in calories - 500 calories or more per drink is not uncommon. Drink 7 of those suckers, and it translates to 1 evil pound.

Can I lose the excess weight? YES - of course I can! A more realistic goal is 1 ½ to 2 pounds per week. Exercise, combined with smart eating, will have me back to my normal weight in about 6 weeks.

It's very easy to put on weight, but it's nearly impossible to lose weight as fast as you can gain weight. Sometimes, life just isn't fair, is it?

By the way, I did succeed and I was sworn off of roasted pig. The coconut rum cake's just a bit harder to kick…

*****

Ken's Overweight Story: Though most of us won't admit such, cops and donuts go hand in hand. Six years ago, I could polish off a six-pack without batting an eye - a six-pack of donuts, that is.

Every morning, our squad congregated in front of a local convenience store. The joint was known for its 'melt-in-your-mouth' donuts, and man were they good!

The place wasn't in the best of neighborhoods, and in the beginning, we had wanted a 'presence' known in the community to deter crime. It worked like a charm. Over the years, the area prospered with new business coming in. I, too,

prospered in body weight, going from a size 36 waist to a size 44 waist. It wasn't pretty, believe me.

I tried passively to lose weight. Did great, too, except for those donuts that faced me every morning.

They were always irresistible and sorta like the old *Lay's Potato Chips* commercials - and I never could eat just one.

Or could I? How addicted to these donuts had I become?

After much thought, I came to a working decision. I would try to allow myself one donut a day as long as I stuck to my diet plan. If I didn't do well on my diet, then I wouldn't be able to have a donut the following day.

On the days that I didn't frequent the store, I'd have another treat.

I'm happy to report that during the 60-pound weight drop, I didn't miss one day without a donut.

Some people might slap my hands; tell me that I haven't got the healthiest diet in the world. Perhaps that's true. However, my last doctor's report made very high marks.

I'm doing the things that I long to do, too, without struggling to do them. Things such as biking, hiking and playing baseball with my kids.

I feel really good about myself. And I feel really good that I'm able to still enjoy the donuts that I love, and maintain my weight and fitness level.

This is a lifestyle that I can certainly live with - and according to my doctor, for a long time to come.

And even though I know that I've got my diet under control, you can never have enough sensible information and motivational support in this area. There is so much hooey out there and it's important to have dependable knowledge at your fingertips.

*****

The above are stories of people who had weight problem and tried various methods that usually fall under standard diet and exercise. Both of these are important for good health and weight maintenance but normally ineffective in losing excess weight and maintain normal weight in the long run. The following are the people who followed the program described in this guide.

9
Here's what Others have to say who followed the Program
(Real names withheld to protect privacy)

"Imagine if your life were a movie and you could just RUN IT BACKWARD!
Make your arteries run clean and clear as a baby's...
Make cancer cells wink out of existence...
Lose weight without dieting...
Make your colon and digestive tract clean...
Melt away arthritis lumps"

Many of the people whose accounts are provided below have experienced these youthful changes and more by following what is described in this book. These techniques are helping people reverse the damage of aging with the miracles of healthy feelings.

Mr. Omkar M wrote: I am 65 years old, vegetarian since past about 15 years and have no major ailments. In Nov 2002 the routine laboratory tests revealed that I have high Cholesterol levels. I was advised to take regular exercise and avoid cholesterol rich diet. After four months I was again tested for lipid profile. There was no significant improvement in cholesterol levels. Hence, the doctor prescribed cholesterol reducing medication which I took till the end of the year 2005. During this period I was in India and got interested in this amazing technique that I followed regularly for about three to four months, the blockage of Arteries is removed 30 to 40 percent and the arteries became clean, making the circulation unimpeded thus preventing heart attack. I started to note improvement and discontinued taking medicines. After about 3 months, my cholesterol levels became low. I weighed less too but **weight** was never a concern for me. Now, my **cholesterol** levels are normal and I do not take any medicine for lowering the cholesterol.

The details of Cholesterol levels during the above period were as under.

Period	Triglycerides	HDL	LDL
Nov 2002	216	37	156
May 2003	212	34	152
Sep 2006	100	44	137

*****

Dr. Pam M reports that my personal experience with the technique has been so profound that I now recommend it to each of my patients. I have observed an increasing ability to achieve balanced health.

I remember one patient who came to me for **menopausal complaints - night sweats, depression, weight problem**, and **chronic constipation**.

During one of her visits, she mentioned that she was considering hypnosis for her negative emotional state. At this point I suggested she practices the technique. As much as I tried to explain to this very intelligent woman, she was 'stuck' on the idea of hypnosis. It was only after I explained the cost-effectiveness; she agreed and is 'free' from her physical and mental problems for the rest of her life.

*****

Ms. Cathrine Larssen says, I used to be regularly bothered by **'acid stomach'** (stress ulcer tendency) and was dependent on medication to relieve this condition. I would have bouts of great pain and require acid-neutralizing medicines to be able to function normally. Since I learned to practice the technique, I have not suffered from this condition. It is completely gone! No medication needed!

I'd also like to add that I have never been as healthy in my entire life as I have been these last three years since started practicing this simple technique. I don't even catch the regular colds anymore!

*****

Despite a successful career and loving friends, I had been extremely **depressed** and very **suicidal** off and on for about four years, says senior sales Executive, Silicon Valley, California. I attempted to avoid the pain by abusing drugs and alcohol, and I developed other addictions including over-eating that made me obese.

After learning the technique, I am glad to be alive. My **drug, alcohol,** and other **addictive behaviors** have all dissolved - not from any therapy ... simply from this simple practice and my **weight** is back to normal.

*****

I began food addiction at age ten and **abused food** for seventeen years, says Janine Hughes, Canonsburg, Pennsylvania. I almost died of **obesity** related complications but still could not stop. I also had many emotional problems, had been in therapy for twenty-three years, and had been through four drug and alcohol treatment centers. This has been a lifelong struggle for me. You can't imagine the continual battle.

I credit this technique for transforming my life and giving me the tools to stay healthy.

*****

I suffered from **Crohn's disease (chronic inflammation of the intestines),** says Gregor Spindler, Liubljana, Slovenia. I was hospitalized for ten days and was treated with Salofalk (3 x 750 mg.)for this gastrointestinal disorder. Two months later I was switched to Madroc, and another two months later I returned to work.

Little over a year after the disease development, I took this simple technique. My physical condition still wasn't particularly good, and 5 month later, I had a second outbreak of the disease and was again hospitalized. Treatment the first two weeks was absolute fasting, with infusion, analgesics, and hydrocortisone. I returned home after four weeks. The doctors proclaimed my treatment to be a miracle, because the prognosis had been 6-8 months of hospital treatment, plus 4-6 months of 'at home care'.

Although I am not yet completely healed, my physical condition is good. Since learning the technique, my health has varied considerably, yet it improves slightly week by week. I believe it may not cure my disease but has kept me comparatively much healthy.

*****

I lost 22 pounds (10 kgs) in 60 days (around 5 kgs in 30 days) doing "*Kapalbhati Pranayam*" 15 minutes in the morning. And also I didn't have to diet for that just that eat healthy, hygienic, says Vivek Mehta.

10

How About Other Popular Banish Your Belly Programs!

There are so many popular banish your belly programs. Some by well educated authors and powerful organizations. Why is this technique so effective! It's a logical thought. However, you will learn that this is nothing like any of those popular programs - you may be familiar with.

Does this quote sound familiar? "This is a fast and easy 15 minute workout that needs no equipment. Pop this video in your VCR/DVD player two or three times a week and you will see a dramatic change in just four weeks. It was developed by Prevention Fitness Editor with Fitness Advisor PhD. The run time is approximately 20 minutes."

I am sure you have heard such claims. You're not alone and there are many such programs from powerful magazines and well known PhD authors. The medical experts suggest that strength training that builds muscle is more effective than cardiovascular exercise to reduce weight. Because more muscle mass burns more calories. I am not saying that it is not true or doesn't work. But you need to be in good shape to carry out these muscle maker programs. People do develop nice muscles and bodies. But with lot more vigorous exercise than you expect, and almost unworkable for someone like me in 60s. I tried many including Prevention VCR in 1990s when I was in fifties. I did not notice a significant difference. And I think that was a good program and good exercises. Even yoga stretches that I do, keep me healthy and flexible but are not as effective as I expect in reducing belly and weight. What I will share does. Even when I am 10 years older and with less physical vigor.

11

Stomach size and its relationship with food Intake

The stomach is a muscular organ - about the size of your hand - that stretches when full and returns to normal when empty. This stretching of the stomach is only temporary. The size of stomach that varies among individuals, affects food intake.

Although bigger people tend to have bigger appetites, the size of the stomach--and not just the size of the body--appears to affect the feeling of fullness, or satiation, during and after a meal, according to research from the Mayo Clinic College of Medicine in Rochester, Minnesota.

The investigators found that compared with normal-weight adults, those who were overweight or obese took longer to feel satiated at mealtime. Similarly, those whose empty stomachs were larger needed more calories to feel completely full.

It was not merely a matter of bigger people having bigger stomachs, said the researchers. Instead, the size of a person's empty stomach (called fasting gastric volume) was related to a feeling of fullness independent of body size.

Their study included 134 healthy volunteers who, after an overnight fast, drank a liquid meal until they reached maximum satiation. Their stomach volume before and after eating was measured through non-invasive imaging. The researchers found that both body mass index (BMI) and fasting gastric volume were independently linked to the time it took participants to become full.

The study suggests that factors governing stomach volume might predispose people to obesity and could serve as targets for weight-control tactics. These control mechanisms could range from eating patterns, such as whether a person eats small meals throughout the day or tends to binge, to hormones, to the nerves that control stomach contraction and relaxation (Gastroenterology, February 2004).

From these studies it is safe to assume that whatever can help reduce the stomach size will help control appetite and thus weight reduction. Further proof is the extreme example of surgical procedure to reduce stomach size. One of the major reasons for surgery to promote weight loss is that the operations close off parts of the stomach to make it smaller. Operations that only reduce stomach size are known as "restrictive operations" because they restrict the amount of food the stomach can hold.

In conclusion, reduced stomach not only improves the appearance but helps control weight. Because, reduced stomach makes you feel full with less food reducing the amount of food eaten and thus the calories consumed. This leads to weight loss. Therefore, you're killing two birds with one-stone, the reduced stomach which reduces weight in this simple but effective exercise.

12

Clean Colon

You may have seen infomercials that sell various ingredients (including cleansing nutrients and chemicals) to cleanse the colon that works wonders and brings weight down. It's true that healthy colon is essential to good health, which makes colon cleansing a must. Everything accumulated in our bowels can be toxic. As these toxins build up, we end up with various diseases, such as being overweight, constipation, digestive problems, Irritable Bowel Syndrome (IBS), Stomach Pain, brain fog, sluggishness/lack of energy, yeast infections. There are so many colon cleansers in the market who like to sell their products at an initial startup cost of $40-$80... Colonix, OxyPowder, Almighty Cleanse, etc.

However, there is almost no information, especially free information that will explain colon cleansing for your health.

Colon Cleansing for Your Health:

So, why do we need colon cleansing? In addition to protruded belly and weight, one word...Toxins.

You see, the colon is one organ that indirectly and directly affects all the other organs in the body. When it's clogged up, the liver for example, can't do its job properly. When the liver can't work efficiently, the kidney suffers, and we notice other ill-effects. So to start curing any symptoms and to get better, we must have clean colon.

The truth is our colon, for most of us, is in an unhealthy state, filled with mucoid plaque, toxins, and a complete mess. Our colon is clogged, leading to constipation. How did we reach this state? Through a combination of a bad diet, lack of exercise, poor lifestyle choices, and bad living conditions.

Take our diet for instance. Most Americans consume too much protein. Protein is necessary, and completely healthy, but too much can lead to over-acidity, which is not good. An overabundance of acid in the body can take a toll on the colon, as it depletes necessary minerals and electrolytes from our body. This then leads to the inability of the colon to tackle harmful bacteria, and toxins.

Many of us not only overeat, but eat foods on a daily basis such as Cookies, cakes, processed foods, chips, sweets, etc. which were not available in nature to be eaten by man. Eating unnatural-processed foods is a big reason why there is mucoid plaque stuck in our colon, and why we all need cleansing our colon.

Harmful chemicals from prescription medication, food, water, air, and pesticides, etc. every single day add toxins to our system, and our immune system has to work overtime to rid our body of these nasty chemicals. This weakening of the immune system leads to a weakening of the colon as well.

Clean Colon provides an alternative method to treat many of our symptoms and problems. It's not just for people with constipation, but for anyone who wishes to feel better, and strengthen their inner organs.

Bowel cleansing is not just about cleansing the colon. It's about indirectly cleansing our small intestines, large intestines, and stomach as well. When we do a cleanse, we are actually cleansing our entire body.

What does our colon do?

The colon consists of the portion of the large intestine that runs from the cecum down to our rectum. The large intestine's purpose is to store waste, reabsorb water, and help maintain electrolyte and water balance. The large intestine does not play any part in actually digesting our food (although bacteria do use the fiber for their own benefit) - that's already done in the small intestine.

How do you know if you have a healthy colon?

Simple, if you have at least one bowel movement a day, with solid bowels, and very little constipation. Of course, if you're a weight-lifter and eat 4000-5000 calories a day, 2 or so bowel movements are normal. But if you're like normal people, you should ideally only have 1-2 bowel movements a day. No more, no less.

So, what do normal bowels look like?

A healthy bowel is 8-12 inches long and around 2.5 inches wide.

The bowels are solid, aren't in little pieces or slimy-like.

Contrary to popular belief, healthy bowels do not have to sink. Or float. Depending on your diet, it can go both ways. Bowel with fruit, vegetables and enough fiber normally floats.

Normal bowels have a brownish color, but a light green color is ok too (unless some kind of food color is consumed).

A normal bowel movement involves absolutely no straining. It's pain-free, and effortless.

Many people who choose to clean their large intestines have constipation problems, marked by constant straining when excreting. This is unhealthy and can lead to other serious illnesses. When constipation occurs, remnants of foods remain inside your body longer than they have to, which is dangerous. Think about this: What happens when you leave a peeled banana outside for several days? It turns rotten. Well, you can imagine why this could cause problems inside your body.

Even if you don't have constipation, colon cleansing can help anyone, especially older people.

We routinely clean our furniture, our toilets, our cars, and the like. Why? To get rid of junk that accumulates. Our body essentially works the same way. Junk, in the form of waste along with toxins accumulates and burdens our major organs such as our large intestine. When our intestine is clogged, we can't absorb necessary nutrients. Toxins circulate back to our body, causing autoimmune diseases such as acne. Cleansing our bowels is a way of maintaining a clean, efficient body.

What does cleansing involve?

Colon cleansing, typically involves a commercial product such as Colonix, or a natural recipe consists of taking a fiber-shake once a day, gradually working up to 3-5 times a day for 2-4 weeks. People usually do a quick fast beforehand, it's not necessary. During the cleanse it is important not to overeat, and not to consume any junk food.

There are people who choose to cleanse with a colon cleanser. There are many in the market right there. The most popular ones are Colonix, OxyPowder, and Dual Action Cleanse. Startup supply may cost between $40 to $80. These claim Colon Cleansing as a simple 3-8 week process that doesn't require any drastic diet changes, or a complete fast. Those who try claim to heal acne, candida, brain fog, digestive problems, and sluggishness. By the end of the regimen, most will feel the difference and feel livelier due to the removal of toxins, healthier bowels, no constipation, and faster transit times. Some people actually even use it to lose weight, since it's so effective in doing that.

How effectively these cleansing agents work? Do these add any more toxins to your system? You don't need to worry.

The techniques in this book are not only free, but are the most natural way to cleanse your colon, and at the same time banish your stomach and bring the weight down.

13

Time to *Kapalbhatise*

It's really amazing how simple things practiced regularly place our mental and physical being to a mind-boggling 'healthy' level. I had been writing about alternate health techniques and use both western scientific and eastern ancient techniques including yoga, breathing, and spirituality in my books. But I have never come across such a doable form of technique involving breathing/yoga that makes perfect scientific sense. Most of yoga that I have come across is either too complicated or too time-consuming. Because of the practicality of *Kapalbhati* technique, I instantly developed a liking for it. Most of us are familiar with or have heard of two forms of *pranayam* (breathing techniques), one is *kapalbhati pranayam* and the other one is the regular *pranayam* (or whatever you call it). And believe me; it works wonders, not only for me but for a whole lot of people who have practiced this sincerely. The good thing about it is, it is short and it gives instant results - skeptics might note that. Now how does it work?

"Sitting in any comfortable or yogic *Padmasana* position, or sitting in chair, or even standing and lying down I begin taking short breaths in and out, exhaling forcefully each time I breathe out, moving my belly in and out in synchronization with my breathing, concentrating on my navel. So, this is not only a breathing exercise, but also an abdominal one. As one practices, one begins to get more in control, the mind concentrating on the navel as it goes in and out. Finally, with more practice, one begins doing it automatically, setting the mind free to roam with the spirit being woken within. This *Pranayam* is done for 10 – 15 minutes, taking rest in between (detailed technique later). "

The other *pranayam* is, as I said, the regular one, where you just need to exhale and inhale alternately to your full lung capacity.

While both of these *pranayams* help overcome blues, negativity, stress and depression, *kapalbhati*, which is also a good abdominal exercise, has this added advantage of bringing your weight to the ideal level. Even a flat-tummied guy like me got rid of 0.5 inch of waistline in two months.

All it takes is 10-15 minutes of my 'precious' time, most of which is wasted in gossip or other unnecessary chores. So folks, if you really want to feel good and look good, go have fun with *kapalbhati,* that is modified and made simple to be done by anyone, at any age, at anytime, and at any place. Am I sounding like a salesman? Neah. I am just sharing my experience. If you can afford to spend your time reading my book and surfing the internet, you can definitely afford to spend 15 minutes of your daily-time for your health.

> *"You know why laughter is the best medicine?*
> *Because it is nothing but a simulation of kapalbhati pranayam."*

Kapalbhati does more than reducing the weight and stomach size, which are almost like excellent side effects (Just as Viagara's side effects to overcome Erectile Dysfunction). *"Kapalbhati"* is also called mind-detoxification technique or cleansing breath. *Kapalbhati* has a remarkable effect as a de-stressing tool and clearing the mind of negative emotions. In fact, the Sanskrit word *"Kapal"* means the skull (here skull means brain, head and any other organ under the skull) and *"bhati"* means polishing / shining / illuminating. *"Kapalbhati"*, as the name suggests, is a method to make the head "sparkling clean" and devoid of toxins. In other words a healthy mind. *Kapalbhati pranayam* is called *'dharti ki sanjivini'* that means it can cure all diseases of the world, says Swami Ramdev.

Warning: If you're suffering from cardiac problems, nasal obstructions, cold and severe respiratory infection, it is advisable to consult your physician. You should also be careful and start slowly if you suffer from High BP, diabetes, abdominal ulcers or some kind of weakness.

Now for the method – How to do it?

"Pranayama or Pranayam" literally means control of Breath. *"Prana"* is Breath or bio energy in the body. On subtle levels *prana* represents the *pranic* energy responsible for life or life force, and *"ayama"* means control. So *Pranayama* is "Control of Breath". One can control the rhythms of *pranic* energy with *pranayama* and achieve healthy body and mind.

In *kapalbhati pranayam*, the act of inhalation or breathing-in is to be done with normal usual force but the act of exhalation has to be done with as much of force as is at your command. The kind of force you apply during sneezing. In doing so, the abdominal area, also makes inward and outward movements. In short, breathe in normally and breathe out forcefully, so as to influence the organs of the abdominal area. (Considerable force is applied to the *Manipura, Swadhishthana & Muladhara Chakras*. Don't worry and simply ignore, if these chakras don't mean anything to you.) This *Pranayam* should easily be done for **five-minutes**. Persons suffering from acute and chronic diseases must practice it for 15 minutes or more as per the capability.

First assume the correct posture (*Asan*). If you cannot comfortably remain in the Lotus Pose (*Padam-asan*), get into an easy position (*Siddh-asan or Sukh-asan*) where you can sit comfortably for a long time. You can sit on a chair or you can do the breathing exercises even lying down on your back with right hand over the chest and left over the belly. You can also do it while standing, if necessary. Remember to open your belt, unhook your bra, loosen your girdle or tie if you happen to be wearing any of these items. Keep the spine straight, with hands on knees. The thumb and index-finger touching as shown below and other three fingers straight. Palm, preferably facing upward. See illustrations below for correct positions.

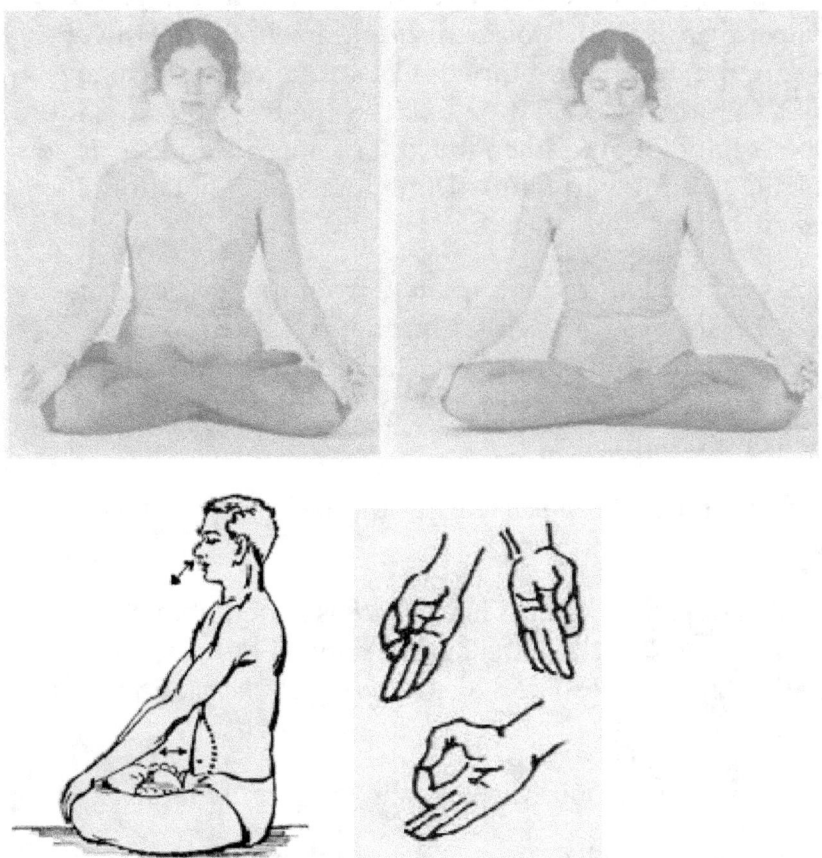

Although, the *kappalbhati pranayam* is remarkably simple, it is important that it is done properly. This *pranayam* is a little different from other kinds of *pranayam*, where *Puraka* (inhalation) and *Rechak* (exhalation) are done with the same amount of force. In *Kapalbhati* more attention is to be given to the act of forceful *Rechak* (exhalation) in which stomach and diaphragm are vigorously applied.

After you acquire a comfortable position with spine erect, breathe normally for about a minute. Once composed, you can begin. First, Exercise the diaphragm by exhaling suddenly and quickly through both nostrils, producing a "puffing" sound. Push air forcefully out. Stomach should itself go in. However, make sure the diaphragm moves upward and stomach goes in during this forceful exhalation. To test the force of exhalation; keep your hand about 6-inch in front of nostrils and see if you feel the air striking you palm. Don't focus on inhalation. It will be automatic and passive.

The air is exhaled almost completely from the lungs with a sudden, vigorous stroke while simultaneously drawing inwards the abdominal muscles. The breath should be expelled fully. Inhaling is automatic - the abdominal muscles will relax automatically.

A cycle or rotation of *Kapalbhati* should be performed as follows :

Inhale and start performing *Kapalbhati* as stated above. That means a strong *Rechaka* (exhalation), natural *Puraka* (inhalation/inspiration) and again strong *Rechaka* and natural *puraka*.

Keep on doing this rotation swiftly in rhythmic manner.

Perform as many cycles as possible and then keep breathing gradually.

This exercise can be done starting with 30 cycles/rotations or 1 minute, increase up to 5 minutes minimum, and up to 10 minutes maximum. A little rest can be taken in between the rounds as convenient. Throughout the exercise, the chest should be kept still without expansion or contraction. Only the diaphragm and stomach muscles are used for *kapalbhati pranayam* and not the upper chest.

Duration and Benefits:

Do this *Pranayam* at the start for a period of three minutes and gradually increase it to five minutes. Initially, if you feel tired in between, take rest for a while and resume. After practice of about two months, you will be able to perform this *Pranayam* for five minutes at a stretch without any fatigue. This is the minimum total duration for which it should be done. In the beginning, you may feel a little pain in the back or abdomen. But this will disappear after some practice. So do not give up.

These are traditional recommendations. However, it can be done for any duration of time starting with 1 minute and increase to any amount of time depending upon your physical condition and your goal towards reducing weight and other health benefits. Do it anytime and anywhere you feel the need to do it. That's what makes it effective and different from traditional techniques. More later on why the technique given here works better than done as usual breathing exercise.

Wondering what this amazingly simple method can do, in addition to weight and stomach reduction, for you? Read on...

The heat generated has POWERFUL effects on the respiratory system as it purifies the nasal passage and the lungs. Even in cases of asthma, it removes spasm in bronchial tubes.

Kapalbhati works wonders on the mind – you will feel totally de-stressed and should experience a unique calmness with this process. The mind becomes remarkably clear. Regular practice will lead you to higher levels of awareness.

The physical benefits include a tremendous stimulation of the digestive organs and the circulatory system. This technique increases exchange of gases in the lungs manifold. There is large-scale elimination of Carbon dioxide and a huge absorption of oxygen.

Do this technique regularly (once or twice or whenever you need it during the day to increase energy) and you'll be truly amazed at the results of this purification method. It is really one of the only methods to really clear the mind of toxins and negative emotions.

"Kapalbhati Pranayam" is known to provide several benefits, according to Swami Ramdev, that can be summarized.

a. Obesity, diabetes, flatulence, constipation, acidity, diseases pertaining to kidneys and prostate gland etc. are cured.

b. If done regularly for five minutes daily, it cleanses the colon while relieving constipation, Blood sugar becomes normal and weight in the abdominal region reduces considerably. Blockages in the arteries are also cleared.

c. Diseases related to *Kapha* like asthma, respiratory troubles, allergies, sinus, etc. are cured. Croesus (liver), hepatitis B, uterus, stomach problems, cholesterol, snoring, concentration, even cancer and AIDS, and various diseases of heart, lungs and brain get cured, says Swami Ramdev.. the 21st century modern guru whose blessings are sought by India's elite, including its vice president, several Supreme Court judges and other senior government officials and politicians.

d. Organs in the abdominal cavity viz. stomach, pancreas, liver, spleen, intestine, prostrate and kidney function more efficiently and develop immunity towards diseases. This is the best exercise; benefits accrued by this cannot be obtained by other *asanas*. It strengthens the intestines and improves digestion.

e. Face become Lustrous and attractive.

f. Peace and stability of mind are achieved. No negative thoughts occur. Troubles like depression are cured.

These are long-term benefits if you follow this breathing exercise in traditional manner. We are presenting this exercise to have more effective impact on stomach and weight loss. But at the same time could be done by anyone irrespective of physical health and age for numerous health benefits.

Finally take a vow [*Shiva Sankalpa*] at the time of performing Kapal-Bhati:
While doing this *Pranayama* think that while exhaling you are throwing all the diseases out of your body. Individuals with mental aberrations like anger, greed, self-ego attachment etc. should develop a feeling of throwing out all the negative and injurious elements along with the air exhaled. In this way the feeling of getting rid of diseases while exhaling imparts a special benefit to the individual.

When to Do it:

For maximum benefits, do the practice regularly, at least twice a day. This technique should better be done on an empty stomach or at least 2 hours after eating. But other times work fine for quick pick up.

This is what I do at least twice to a count of 30 or 1 minute to 5 minutes each time. Total of about 15 minutes or more in entire day. I do it anytime for any length, at any place just like taking a break to relax. This is the beauty of this technique where it differs from regular *kapalbhati* or other rigid programs as explained in next section:

a. I do it in the morning, while lying in the bed with right hand on chest and left hand on belly

b. Before breakfast in sitting position

c. In the after noon when sluggish either sitting in chair, standing or lying down.

d. At night when lying down.

e. Even before eating or when hungry

f. Any other time of day whenever feel the need to do it, sitting, standing, lying down, or even walking to a count of 30.

14

What's so different about the *Kapalbhati* Technique that Works

The difference is joy, simplicity, effectiveness, and convenience that you can find in this technique. There is no where you can go wrong in *kapalbhati* technique. Think for a moment. We replace stale air with fresh oxygen. We focus on breathing and do kind of meditation. We exercise our abdominal muscles. And why wait for a specific place or specific posture or specific time to do these good acts. Why not do anytime anywhere-- sitting down, lying down, standing up, while taking a walk, and so on. And why need specific repetitions. Do 10 times, 20 times, 30 times, 40 times or up to whatever number you're comfortable with. Then increase at your own pace.

What we recommend is as simple as taking break regularly from whatever you do. But as human beings we normally look for some sort of procedure, which is clearly spelt out by some guru or by some organization or some *ashram*. I have followed the method described here and have greatly benefited from it, which is the reason of my excitement to share with you. I have attained in weeks in terms of weight and waste size what I could not achieve in years.

We should, initially, set aside one or two (say ten to fifteen minutes) periods within a twenty-four hour period strictly to learn the technique and make it a routine. *Kapalbhati*, of course, can be combined with any other exercise. For example, with meditation, with other breathing exercises, jogging, walking, and various sports. Do *Kapalbhati* regularly and give it prominence in your daily living. Get yourself into a routine. It will be difficult in the beginning, but once you establish a pattern you will find great joy in it. Most of us use morning or evening for using different techniques to improve our physical and mental health. In a busy life in which time - management is very important, my personal recommendation is to use anytime of the day as I do in my routine.

Go through the routine you set down and go back to sleep and get up at the usual time that you wake up to face the world for the day! The sleep that one has after doing *kapalbhati* is the most blissful and restful. If you suffer from insomnia, I guarantee that this procedure will help you.

If any recommendation is not practical due to your circumstances then be practical - as long as you do develop a daily routine. Some precautions: Many 'gurus' and 'training centers' advocate various methods of breathing that may include *kapalbhati*. Some of them consider it more of a cleansing exercise called *shuddhi-kriya* and may not even include it. Some will prescribe special postures, penances, dressing, clothing, colors to follow strictly. Generally, all will tell you how hard these techniques are and that theirs is the only true method.

There is nothing secretive and strict about *kapalbhati* as long as it produces the results and your health allows you to do it without any harm to your body. There are, of course, genuine basic procedures that we need to follow.

All we have to do is to make a sincere effort to follow a regular daily routine. Though proper weight is a serious health concern, to achieve this way is fun. It is a very joyful experience - give yourself a chance to experience this joy! Secondly, remember that we have to focus our mind on the procedure when we do *kapalbhati*. The purpose is lost if our mind is involved in our mundane, daily problems.

It is also a good idea to get together some like-minded friends and do *kapalbhati* once in a while (say, weekly) and also talk about it and encourage each other. In short, create an atmosphere which is conducive to keep up and enjoy at the same time. Make it a habit to keep yourself RELAXED and upright. If you try too hard in the early stages you will lose the sense of joy and it will become like a work.

If you experience a discomfort initially, all that is happening is that you are trying too hard, RELAX! Remember, *kapalbhati* is JOY, not a job, and definitely not hard work. Concentrating too hard is natural. Just like learning how to ride a bicycle. Because you are tensed and trying too hard, you keep falling off the bike but, with time, as you relax and become flexible, you will ride the bicycle with ease and enjoy the ride. Similarly, relax and any kind of discomfort will be gone.

There are adverse forces which will try everything negative to discourage you - that is their job in the "Order of Things". Do not allow these dark forces to stop you from the 'purpose of your one-life' which is ultimately to live in the best of your health. Our natural state of existence is health, not disease.

Let the joy and ecstasy linger on for the rest of the day. In today's fast un-natural lifestyle it will help you keep not only at proper weight but healthy. It raises your self esteem, puts you in a state of confidence, and everything positive which brings you success in life. You will realize your full potential and reach your aspirations in this life

15

How does It Work for Weight Loss!

Here're the simple reasons that it works for weight loss:

1. When the stomach is exercised by abdominal movements, you feel less hungry. So you feel satisfied by simply eating less. Also the reduced stomach size means less food consumption. Abdominal flab lost in this manner doesn't return easily and you remain happy and young for a long time. Hence *kapalbhati* is definitely a smarter way to look sexy and stay healthy.

2. *Kapalbhati* is NOT a typical *Pranayama* exercise, it is a Cleansing Technique, also known as *shuddhi-kriya*. The elimination of waste in the digestive system means reduced weight and elimination of toxins. Waste can be several pounds depending upon the digestive health of a person.

3. People normally eat when they lack energy/ sluggish/ bored. The breathing involved in *kapalbhati pranayam* increase energy by increasing oxygen intake. This not only provides energy and stimulates metabolism but also burn more calories in addition to curving the appetite.

As you force the cells of your body to produce energy during breathing exercise as happens in aerobic exercise, the tiny sub-cellular sites of energy production (called mitochondria) are encouraged to become more efficient and also actually to increase in number. Breathing exercise combined with proper nutrition, "tunes up" mitochondrial function and increases the ability to clear fat from the body. Aerobic exercise alters chemistry, and increases metabolic rate. All of these cause you to burn more calories even when asleep.

4. *Kapalbhati* as the name indicates clears your head from tensions and depression. So it saves those who eat to fight depression or similar problems. One of the factors that influence overweight is the psychosocial aspects of over-eating; people experience frustration, depression, worry, guilt, shame, hopelessness, isolation and unusual stress which often lead them to seek compensation in eating.

5. I often do *kapalbhati* before eating even when waiting for a food, for a count of 30 or so. This helps from over-eating. Even if I feel hungry during the day, I do *kapalbhati* and many times the desire to eat diminishes leaving me lighter. I don't run for a snack if it is close to dinner time, I do *kapalbhati*. Experiment with your own situation and notice what makes a difference for you. It's fun.

6. The fact is, *Kapalbhati* is highly energizing abdominal breathing exercise that burns calories. Rapid movement of abdominal muscles in and out is very good exercise to get rid of the accumulated fats in the abdominal region. Despite what you may think, you are not doomed by bad genes passed to you from your parents – by doing *Kapalbhati*, you can learn to work with your genes and not against them, to automatically boost your metabolism.

16

Supplemental Exercises to Boost Energy

The supplemental exercises are purely to boost energy, and I will highly recommend that you do these. These may not be considered mandatory for reducing belly or to lose weight, although these will help toward that goal. I do use them, especially deep breathing and alternate nostril breathing.

The importance of *Prana* or the breath as an instrument to control diseases is recognized universally. In fact, no life is possible without breathing. Breathing may be considered as the most important of all the functions of the body for indeed all the other functions depend on it. *Prana* (Chi) is thus rightly called the life force energy and the art of modification of normal form of *prana* through its conscious control is known as *pranayama* (Control of Breath). In view of its importance, the Yogis from times immemorial have emphasized on the need of regular practice of *Pranayama* for harmony of body, mind and spirit. *Pranayama* is the fourth limb of the eightfold Yoga system founded by Maharishi Patanjali and is capable of addressing all kinds of physical and mental ailments effectively.

The exercises given here are scientifically developed and redesigned. These are comprised of seven well known *pranayama* techniques of Maharishi Patanjali and are recommended by modern guru Swami Ramdev:

1. ***Bhastrika Pranayam*** (Deep Breathing) for 3 to 5 minutes

(I do in 4 cycles, counting 30 each time then relax and continue with the next cycle.)

2. ***Kapalbhati Pranayam*** (Rapid Exhalation Breathing) 5 to 10 minutes

(I do in 10 cycles, counting 30 each time then relax and continue with the next cycle.)

3. ***Bahya Pranayam*** (Holding Breath) using three *bandhs* (Physical Locks) for 2 minutes (I do 3-5 times applying three bandhs and relaxing in between)

4. ***Anulom- Vilom Pranayam*** (Alternate-nostril Breathing) 5 minutes

(I do in 10 sets of cycles, counting 30 each time then relax and continue with the next set.)

5. ***Bhramari Pranayam*** (Meditational Breathing) 2 minutes (minimum of 3 cycles)

(I do 3-5 times while closing eyes and focusing on *Ajna chakra* (forehead between eyes known as third eye) and relaxing in between)

6. ***Udgeet Pranayam*** ('OM' Chanting Breathing) 5 times

(I do 5 times while focusing on *Ajna chakra* and relaxing in between)

7. ***Ujjayi Pranayam*** (Throat Breathing) 3 to 11 cycles.

(I do 3 times while glottis held partially closed during inhaling)

A regular practice of these techniques for about twenty minutes as briefly explained in the following paragraphs, guarantees maintenance of good health and healing from hypertension, over weight problems, diabetes to serious and even chronic ailments. It also works as a prophylactic to ward off future ailments. The results for those who practice are simply amazing.

1. BHASTRIKA PRANAYAM (Deep Breathing)

Bhastrika Pranayam involves movement of the belly using diaphragm. In this *pranayam*, equal emphasis is laid on exhalation and inhalation.

Sit in a meditative posture (*Asana*) like *Sukh Asana* (cross – legged) or on a chair with your spine straight and inhale filling the lungs up to the diaphragm and exhale with full force emptying the lungs. Do it with a rhythm. Repeat the cycle. The inhalations and exhalations should be done with slow speed or medium speed or fast speed depending on your practice, capacity and state of health. Those having weak heart or week lungs should do *Bhastrika* with slow speed. This *pranayam* should be done for a minimum of 2 minutes to a maximum of 5 minutes. (I do in 4 cycles, counting 30 each time then relax and continue with the next cycle.) For better results, you may also simultaneously visualize that the divine power, energy, joy and peace entering your body through the process of breathing during these exercises.

2. KAPALBHATI PRANAYAM (Rapid Exhalation Breathing)

It's mostly repetition of what has been described earlier in detail. The modifications that work are the main aim of this book. *Kapalbhati* which means shining skull or forehead , is considered one of the most important techniques. *Kapalbhati* is also done in the same easy sitting posture, the whole attention is given to only exhalation and no effort is applied to inhale. However, breath is allowed to be inhaled in quantity that one would have drawn in a natural course.

Sit in a convenient posture and without consciously breathing in; breathe out with full force during exhalation, simultaneously ensuring contraction of abdomen muscles with each exhalation. Repeat the process of exhalations without deliberate inhalations as long as you can. The minimum time allotted to this *pranayama* is 5 minutes which can be increased to a maximum of 10 minutes with a short break for rest in between, if necessary. (I do in 10 cycles, counting 30 each time then relax and continue with the next cycle. Also do 2 more cycles: one after the *Anulom-Vilom Pranayam* and other after the *Bhramari Pranayam.*) While breathing out, one should visualize that all the diseases and toxins are being thrown out with each exhalation.

Highly effective in controlling obesity, diabetes, kidney and prostate problems, heart, brain and lung problems and many other diseases; this technique increases the glow on the face of the practitioner.

3. *BAHYA PRANAYAM* (Holding Breath using physical locks called *Bandhs*)

Bahya pranayam is marked by suspension or retention or holding the breath after exhalation of breath and applying *mahabandh.* A *Mahabandh* (a *bandh* stands for a physical lock to control the flow of *prana*) is comprised of three bandhs, namely *Jalandhur Bandh* (touching the chin on the pit located near the base of throat); *Uddiyan Bandh* (pulling the stomach in so as to touch the back)) and *Mul bandh* (pulling up the perineum by contracting the anus and tightening of the lower abdomen). In *Mahabandh,* all these three *bandhs* are applied together.

Remain seated in one of the meditative postures, first breathe in and fill your lungs up to diaphragm and then breathe out with full force and suspend the breathing process, simultaneously applying the *mahabandh.* Maintain this position till you feel like inhaling again. Now inhale releasing the three *bandhs* gradually starting with *Jalandhur Bandh* and ending with *Mul Bandh*. This completes one cycle of *bahya pranayam*. A minimum of three such cycles are recommended which take two minutes to complete. While doing this *pranayam* also do not forget to visualize that all your diseases and toxins are being thrown out with each exhalation.

4. *ANULOM-VILOM PRANAYAM* (Alternate-nostril Breathing)

This *pranayam* is done with alternate breathing from the left and right nostrils for cleansing of *Nadis* (energy meridians).

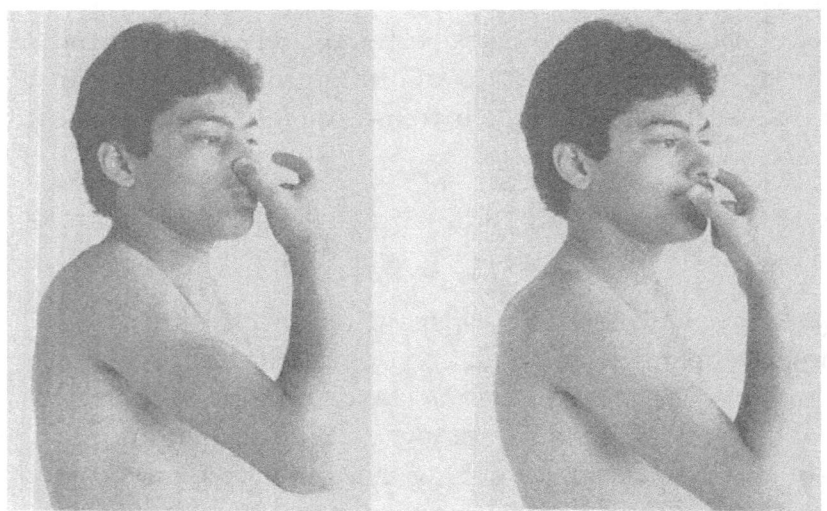

Seated in a convenient posture, start off with slow inhalation from the left nostril by closing the right nostril with the right hand thumb, and after fully filling the lungs, breathe out slowly from the right nostril by closing the left nostril with forefinger (or third and fourth finger, if more convenient) of right hand. Now breathe in from the right nostril with closed left nostril in the above manner and exhale from the left nostril by closing the right nostril with the right thumb. It completes one cycle. Continue cycles of alternate breathing for 5 to 10 minutes with break for rest after each minute, if required. (I do in 10 sets of cycles, counting 30 each time then relax and continue with the next set.) Gradually, with practice, the speed of breathing can be increased to medium and to fast. While you do this *pranayam* visualize that the Divine power and the Divine knowledge is being bestowed upon you in the process. The practice of this pranayama for 5 minutes a day will result in activation of the *Muladhar Chakra* (Root *Chakra* or energy center) causing the arousal of *Kundalini* power (dormant serpentine power located on the root *chakra*). The arousal of *Kundalini* power results from the arousal of *Sushumna nadi* (the central energy meridian) as a consequence of repeated rubbing and churning of the breath in the *Ida* (left meridian) and *Pingla* (right meridian) *Nadis*.

The practice of *Anulom-vilom* for a period of three to four months can open up thirty to forty percent of the heart arteries' blockages. This pranayam alleviates all the diseases of the body, leads to the state of joy, enthusiasm for living, fearlessness, peace of mind and deep meditation.

5. *BHRAMARI PRANAYAM* (Meditational Breathing)
 Bhramara means a bumble bee. The *Pranayam* gets its name from the resounding sound produced like the bumble bee, during exhalation.

Close both ears with your thumbs (pushing tragus-small projection just in front of the ear opening), place index fingers on both sides of the forehead, place the rest three fingers each on both sides of the nose, and keep the mouth closed. Now breathe in fully. Slightly pressing the sides of the nose with the fingers, exhale from both the nostrils, as if chanting 'OM' from the nose, making a humming sound like a bee. The noise should reverberate through the entire body. Repeat the exercise five to 11 times or do it for about 2 minutes. You will quite enjoy this *pranayam* which will relax you and activate all the glands of the head.

This *Pranayam* activates the *Ajna chakra* (considered third eye energy center) which is part of forehead between the two-eyes. Always focus on *Ajna Chakra* while chanting 'OM'. This puts you in touch with the divine element within you.

6. *UDGEET PRANAYAM* ('OM' Chanting Breathing)
  'OM' has a universal sound. Chant 'OM' (long au and short m) loudly. Take a deep breath and release the breath through the mouth making the sound 'OM'. Repeat this five to 11 times.

It brings you in meditative state and helps insomnia patients to get sleep.

7. *UJJAYI PRANAYAM* (Throat Breathing)
This requires drawing air in through both nostrils with the glottis held partially closed. *Ujjayi* translates as "what clears the throat and masters the chest area." This partial closure of the glottis produces a sound like that heard in sobbing, except that it is continuous and unbroken. The sound should have a low but uniform pitch and be pleasant to hear. Friction of air in the nose should be avoided; consequently no nasal sounds will be heard. A prolonged full pause should begin, without any jerking, as soon as inhalation has been completed. Hold the breath using chin lock. Prolong the pause as long as possible. Exhale smoothly and slowly through left nostril while closing the right nostril with right hand thumb. When properly performed, exhalation proceeds slowly and steadily through the left nostril with the glottis partially closed as in inhalation. Exhalation should be complete. Repeat 3 to 11 times.

Ujjayi gets rid of the phlegm. It helps cure the snoring and thyroid problems.

Hint: If you feel tense during any of the exercises: relax by breathing in deeply through the nose and then breathe out through the mouth with a relaxing sound of Ahhhh.

After completing all the seven breathing exercises, relax for some time in *Savasana* (Corpse posture) with normal breathing keeping the eyes closed, lying down on the back keeping some distance between the legs and spreading the hands away from the body.

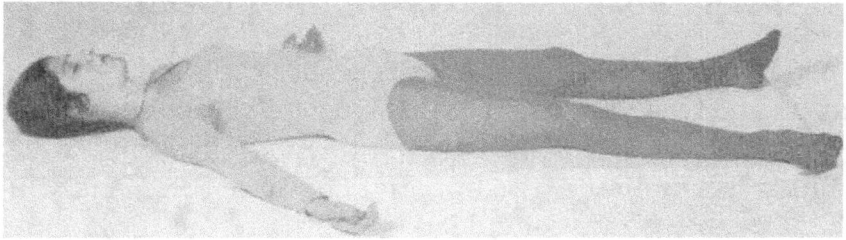

These *Pranayama* exercises offer multiple benefits. It addresses the diseases of the chest, heart, and brain. Highly effective in controlling diabetes, migraine, gastric problem, hypertension, constipation, allergy, kidney diseases, even chronic diseases like cancer, a regular practice of the seven techniques of the package promises to improve immunity to diseases, detoxify the body, bring a glow on the face, improve eyesight and save the practitioner from stress and depression. One can achieve spiritual power due to activation of the *chakras* (body energy centers) in the process which results in arousal of the dormant serpentine energy known as *Kundalini*, the power of which is simply spectacular.

PART III

17

Science behind Success of this program

We already know that any stomach exercise program reduces stomach and controls weight. This is just one part of the program. The second point is that proper use of specific breathing techniques is very important for its success, and you will realize the science behind it.

We breathe in air that contains life-giving-oxygen. The oxygen from air comes into close contact with blood in the lungs. The blood carries oxygen to every cell of the body and the cells utilize the oxygen for energy production through metabolic activities. So better the oxygen supply, higher the metabolism, and better the energy production by burning more calories. Many people do not know the effective use of breathing, cheating their bodies of the very oxygen that boosts energy production and burn calories.

18

Boosting Energy Production and Burning Calories

An average adult breathes more than 12,000 quarts of air a day. This is not only body's largest intake of any substance, but the most immediately important to life. The life giving component of air is oxygen, with minute amount of several other inert gases. More than half of our body weight is oxygen (water is eight-ninth oxygen).

We need oxygen to burn food (calories) and release energy by the process of respiration (synonym for breathing) that goes on incessantly in everyone of our billions of body cells. Cells use oxygen and produce carbon dioxide in their vital activities. The one must be supplied continuously, the other removed, else living machinery comes to a halt in a very short time period. However, cells do not inhale or exhale or breathe in the ordinary sense. Billions of internal cells are in fact shut off from direct contact with an oxygen rich atmosphere. An efficient means of bringing oxygen from the outside world to every cell, and of removing carbon dioxide, is primarily carried by the action of chest and lungs, which are the vital components to carry the process of breathing that in turn provides vital energy and burn calories which otherwise may store as fat and thus excess weight.

Breathing is one of the ancient techniques in the east, which is practiced to achieve perennial youth and immortality and a method to achieve enlightenment in Buddhism, especially the Zen sect. In the modern society breathing and aerobics are becoming the most popular exercises to maintain not only proper weight but to achieve the total well-being.

The energy supplied by the respiratory process affects the functioning of our brain, our stamina, and our basic physical well-being. Biologically, the process of respiration involves a series of chemical reactions that are completed through two major path-ways, **glycolysis** and **Krebs** cycle. The major purpose of these series of reactions is to provide energy along with waste carbon dioxide and water by burning food in the presence of oxygen.

FOOD + OXYGEN $\rightarrow$ ENERGY + CARBON DIOXIDE + WATER

The proteins, fats, and carbohydrates from food are broken down in the process of digestion; they yield amino acids, fatty acids, and simple sugars, respectively. These products are then absorbed into the blood, either directly into the intestinal capillaries or indirectly by the lymphatic system, as in the case of fats and triglycerides. Upon absorption the food, whatever its origin, must be handled in one of two ways. The first priority is to satisfy energy requirements of the moment, and secondly food not required immediately is placed in storage for later use. Oxygen, which must be present for producing energy, cannot be stored for later use, so our survival depends on a steady supply from breath to breath.

The cells of our body are energy factories, so to speak. In our cells through the process of oxidation, fuels coming from the food that has been eaten or from stored fat are turned into energy in the presence of oxygen. The process completes through a series of reactions and produces energy (by combining ADP and phosphate to reform the energy-rich compound ATP) along with waste carbon dioxide and water. This energy captured by the ATP (adenosine triphosphate) molecule powers the various biological functions of the body. It is important to realize that the oxygen delivery system is a continuous dynamic process which must continue from breath to breath, whereas the fuel transport system can rely on storage for satisfying our needs from minute to minute. This explains why a person can fast for long periods of time but cannot hold a breath more than about one minute. Because the delivery and utilization of oxygen are crucial with respect to energy/metabolism; the breath that provides oxygen is often called **vital breath** or **vital energy** or *prana*.

We constantly drain our life force or vital energy by our thinking, willing, acting or motion of muscles. On going involuntary functions of the body such as heart beat and digestion is using energy day and night, whether we are awake or asleep. Since all these activities use up the life force, constant replenishing is necessary, which can be accomplished primarily through breathing that produces energy and burn calories.

19

Energy without Vigorous Exercises

We are born with fixed number of breaths!
When that number is used, the death happens!!
A legend from Eastern traditions

People following a program of breathing exercises not only boost metabolism and burn more calories but show a lower rate of breathing per minute. The amount of air breathed per minute increases due to more amount of air inhaled per breath. This is due to effective use of diaphragm in those who practice breathing exercises. For example, those engaged in breathing exercises have an average of 6 breaths per minute as compared to a normal person with 14 to 18 breaths per minute and the amount of air breathed per minute of 12 liters as compared to 7 liters in normal healthy individuals. This means that the amount of air per breath increases from 0.5 liter in normal individuals to 2 liters per breath in those taking breathing practices. The breathing exercises boost metabolism by substantially increasing the volume of oxygen supplied to and the volume of carbon dioxide extracted from the body.

Physical exercise (especially aerobics) is another way of increasing the amount of breathed air, and in well-conditioned athletes, the air intake may increase to 160 liters per minute, or even more in response to short-term maximum metabolic demands. However, the breathing exercises as compared to strenuous physical exercises have the advantage of providing energy without physical exertion and can be done irrespective of age or physical condition. Moreover, breathing exercises teach the full utilization of the lungs, emphasizing depth rather than rate of breathing.

In general most people breathe in a shallow manner and use their lungs at less than one-third of their full capacity. To correct this, breathing that uses the respiratory system to its optimum potential is required, letting as much oxygen into the body as possible while removing as much waste carbon dioxide as possible.

There are people everywhere who consciously or unconsciously have control over the vital breath or energy. These spiritualists, mind healers, scientists, hypnotists or simply outstanding individuals in any sphere of life perhaps stumbled on the discovery of vital energy without knowing its nature. However, the vital energy can be used consciously, because breathing functions both automatically (like flow of blood or the beat of heart or digestion of food) and voluntarily (like the movement of hands or blinking of eyes). It is the controllable nature that enables us change the rate and tidal volume of our breath to meet the needs of our body.

In the practice of breathing, the mind plays a great role and it is important to observe consciously everything that takes place in the process of breathing. The pleasant situation as opposed to unpleasant results in deep breathing whereas anger and anxiety has dramatically opposite effects and results in shallow breathing.

We know that deep breathing has a calming effect on the whole personality, reducing jumpiness and nervous tension. Shallow, poor breathing causes anxiety, depression, loss of energy and chronic fatigue. In addition to good health, deep breathing enhances feminine beauty. It burns undesirable fat, makes the skin smooth and glowing, produces a flawless complexion, and puts a bright sparkle in the eyes. A common application of learned deep breathing in the western world are the pregnant women who are taught certain types of breathing exercises for natural less painful childbirth. Deep breathing can be valuable to alcohol, smoke and other drug addicts, since the exercises tend to normalize the various organs, glands, and nervous system.

People take drugs such as heroin because it gives them comfort by stimulating the production of endorphin. Studies on respiration have indicated that practice of deep breathing stimulate endorphin production in the blood. The increased level of endorphin results in maintaining mental and physical comfort. Practice of breathing exercises boost energy production, and can help the drug addicts avoid the use of dangerous toxic drugs and overweight to avoid excessive indulgence in food.

The correct habit of breathing, along with a natural diet and health care, can regenerate people for whom the modern problems of civilized man, such as blood pressure, heart diseases, asthma, chronic stress, sleeplessness, and overweight would be only medical names in the dictionary. Deep rhythmic breathing cannot only prolong our lives, but can keep us vital and youthful even in senior years. In addition to the physical benefits derived through breathing, use of correct breathing can also increase will power, self-control, power of concentration, moral qualities, and even spiritual evolution.

The importance of breathing can be summarized in the words of a popular yoga teacher Sri Krishnamacharya: "Do the deep breathing whenever you are feeling tired, nervous, tense, hungry, too hot or too cold. Do it when you need extra energy, vitality and strengths or when your hopes are low and your faith failing. Also do it whenever you face addressing an audience, especially an unsympathetic one." He suggested that whenever you address a crowd, first take a few deep breaths and during the last inhalation 'take in' the vibrations of the audience, hold the breath for a few seconds, then exhale with the first spoken word.

Breathing therapy has been practiced secretly for thousands of years in the east, and had been considered an integral part of healthy living. The mechanisms of the breathing therapy involving a conscious straining and relaxing of the muscles and nerves and also the mind through breathing are common practices.

In short, you can achieve total well-being including weight control through breathing practices without vigorous exercises-- a quest which is only a dream for many of us.

20

Weight Control and Breathing/Aerobics

Everybody knows that vigorous aerobic exercises not only improve our heart, lungs, and muscles but is the most effective method for weight control. Clearly, most people accept the proposition that physical exercise results in increased heart activity and greater oxygen consumption; these are the bases for popular aerobics workouts.

The term "aerobics" means "utilizing oxygen" or "living in air." In other words, certain exercises are performed to increase oxygen intake as, for example, running, biking, breathing practices.

Aerobic exercises refer to those activities that require oxygen for prolonged periods and place such demands on the body that it is required to improve its capacity to handle oxygen. As a result of aerobic exercise, there are beneficial changes that occur in the lungs, the heart, and the vascular system. More specifically, regular exercise of this type enhances the ability of the body to move air into and out of the lungs; the total blood volume increases; and the blood becomes better equipped to transport oxygen. Aerobic exercises usually involve endurance activities which don't require excessive speed. In fact, it is better to use long, slow distances than is to rely on short, fast bursts of energy.

The purpose is to increase vital energy, and to strengthen the lungs and heart, whether utilize eastern breathing exercises or western aerobic program or better the combination of both. All this translates to better looking body and normal weight.

Characteristics: Aerobic exercise, in fact, may be a part of daily living, because even when you are reading this book, you are performing exercise in an aerobic steady state. In other words, you are breathing regularly and you will continue inhaling and exhaling air as long as there is life.

The main difference between what you are doing and what a marathoner is doing is that your steady state of energy expenditure is at a level much lower than that of the marathoner. The marathoner will fatigue ultimately, due to the fact that his or her energy expenditure is 12-15 times above your basal or resting rate. And your resting heart and respiratory rates are not operating at a level high enough to place demands on the body, as compared to the runner.

For an exercise to be considered aerobic, according to Western Fitness experts, four things are necessary:

1. It must be a steady, non-stop activity.

2. It must be sustained for a minimum of 12 minutes.

3. It must be at your training heart rate which determines your pace. (Training heart rate is 70-80% of your maximum heart rate. Maximum heart rate is 220 minus your age. For example, the pulse rate during an aerobic exercise should be roughly between 140 to 160 for a person of 20 years of age.)

4. You must exercise at least three or four times per week.

Benefits: Aerobic exercise has become a part of the widespread physical-fitness movement in the developed world including United States. Exercise improves the oxygen delivery by increasing the maximum capacity of the lungs. During exercise, the lungs increase their ability to move air from approximately 7 liters per minute at rest to 100-200 liters per minute during maximum effort. Also the heart can increase its output of blood from 4-6 liters per minute to 20-40 liters per minute at this same maximum effort. Physical stress strengthens the heart (the pump), can help to enlarge the major blood vessels (with high-level endurance training), and can improve the delivery of oxygen to the cells in the muscle group that is being used.

The apparatus for using oxygen in the cells of the exercising muscle are also increased as a result of the training effect. Therefore, with increasing physical fitness with exercise, the ability to utilize oxygen is increased. When you improve the capacity of heart function and blood vessels, there will be continued optimal functioning and survival of all the cells in the body that benefit from a good oxygen delivery system.

Individuals who exercise for endurance-type activities develop enlarged arteries to carry the increased volume from the heart to the capillaries where the exchange of oxygen will take place. This has been shown by autopsies of a marathon runner who was still competing at the time of death and of African Tribesmen whose life style requires long-distance walking or running until they die. The capillaries within an exercised muscle group increase in number, owing to the strain, and they can accept increased blood flow with an enhanced ability to exchange oxygen. The increased ability to deliver and utilize oxygen is not present in muscle groups that have not been exercised. This difference shows in exercise stress testings.

Some of the beneficial effects of aerobic exercise are summarized:

1. The total blood volume increases so that the body is better equipped to transport oxygen-and thus the individual has more endurance when engaging in strenuous physical activities.

2. The capacity of the lungs increases, and some studies have

associated this increase in "vital capacity" with a greater longevity.

3. The heart muscle grows stronger, is better supplied with blood, and with each stroke, the heart can pump more blood (increased stroke volume).

4. The beneficial kind--high-density lipoprotein (HDL) increases, which results in decrease of total cholesterol: HDL ratio, and thus there is a reduction in the person's risk of developing atherosclerosis, or hardening of the arteries. (HDL prevent atherosclerosis by removing cholesterol from artery walls and returning it to the liver for excretion.)

5. The ability to deliver nutrients increases throughout the body via circulatory system and thus more personal energy is felt.

Aerobics and Weight Control: As you force the cells of your body to produce energy during aerobic exercise, the tiny subcellular sites of energy production (called mitochondria) are encouraged to become more efficient and also actually to increase in number. Aerobic exercise, combined with proper nutrition, "tunes up" mitochondrial function and increases the ability to clear fat from the body. Aerobic exercise increases muscle, tones it, alter its chemistry, and increases its metabolic rate. All of these cause you to burn more calories even when asleep.

Overweight is generally the result of energy intake that is greater than energy expanded. The fuel from food and oxygen from breathing create the energy vital to our capacity for work and play. It is important to keep a good balance between the fuel taken into the body and the energy that is spent, so that the unspent fuel (excessive food intake measured in calories) is not converted to fat and accumulate in the body as fat, or adipose tissue. It is believed that the rate of fat deposition is higher in overweight people as compared to those with normal weight (due to the effect of overweight on body physiology). To avoid the fat accumulation that causes overweight is desirable, not only in terms of good looks, but more important, in terms of good health. The problem of overweight is a new one: never before has man had so wide a choice---or so regular a supply---of good food; neither did he has such a common use of vehicles that even a natural exercise such as walking would need special efforts.

Factors which influence overweight and upset the caloric balance may include heredity, endocrine factors, physical activity of an individual, number of fat cells, greater intestinal length, or psychosocial-emotional problems. In the psychosocial aspects of over-eating, people experience frustration, depression, worry, guilt, shame, hopelessness, isolation and unusual stress which often leads them to seek compensation in eating. To prevent an increase in body weight and body fat because of a caloric imbalance, any program of weight control must establish an equilibrium between energy input and energy output by either decreasing the intake of food calories or increasing the energy expenditure by exercise or physical activity.

The statistics indicate that the long-term maintenance of a particular low-calorie diet is extremely difficult. Similarly, increasing energy expenditure through physical activity, while not unpleasant in itself, does require a personal commitment in terms of time and life style that many people are not willing to make. However, a serious aerobic exercise program pursued along with a sensible diet (Dhillon, S.S. 1983. Health, Happiness, and Longevity: Eastern and Western Approach. Japan Publications, Tokyo/Harper & Row, New York.) can tip the balance in favor of our maintaining or losing poundage.

Exercise helps in weight control not only by using up calories directly, but your body burns extra calories for up to fifteen hours afterward. Even at the same weight, an active person looks trimmer than one who is sedentary because muscle tissue has a smaller volume than the same weight of fat. Muscle tissue also uses more calories to sustain itself than does an equivalent amount of fat, so if you are well muscled, you can eat more without gaining than can a person who weighs the same but has a higher percentage of body fat.

The aerobic exercise program may include any of the exercises that will result in aerobic activity as a part of living. For example, walk instead of taking a cab or a bus, use the stairs instead of elevators, help yourself with house chores (gardening, mowing the lawn, washing the car, or shoveling the snow), Play golf without a golf cart, replace power tools and appliances where possible.

These are only some of the examples of activities, which can be kept in mind. Much of this comes from self-observation in the form of daily records, combined with will power and efforts to change small details in one's life style as an investment in long-term weight control.

We know that exercise in any form including aerobics uses energy and will, therefore, burn calories. Moreover, regular exercise in addition to burning off extra calories helps to regulate the appetite, so that one is less likely to consume more calories than the body needs. According to Dr. Kenneth cooper (Aerobics Center, Dallas), exercise before the evening meal (but no earlier than 2 hours prior to the meal) is more effective in losing or controlling body fat and weight. The reason for this appears to be that vigorous exercise not only depresses the appetite but also raises the metabolic rate which otherwise tends to slow down as nighttime approaches.

Aerobic Exercises: There are many aerobic exercises that qualify for an effective aerobics program. You can choose cross-country skiing, swimming, jogging or running, cycling, walking, jumping rope, rowing, roller skating, ice skating, aerobic dancing, jumping jacks, and almost any other activity that will get your heart rate up to a level, where, over a sustained period of time, beneficial changes can take place in your cardiovascular system.

Contrary to what many people think, you do not have to commit your life to marathon competition to get the benefits from an aerobic exercise. Remember, if you run more than 3 miles five times per week (or a combination totaling 15 miles per week), you are running for something other than fitness, such as competition or ego-building. Of course, if you want to go into competition and run in races such as the marathon, then you will need to spend more time with your aerobics activity.

Simple aerobic activity like walking goes beyond weight and cardiovascular function. It soothes nervous tension, relieves anxiety, and eases frustration. Most of all, walking gives us the opportunity to think and relax as we give our body a chance to unwind. Walking after dinner helps to get a good sleep, especially for sedentary workers. But no matter what aerobic activity you choose, pay attention to your breathing. By all means enjoy vigorous aerobic program if your health and age permit it. Many of the breathing exercises, however, are quite effective and can be done at any age.

Warning: Like any exercise program, move slowly. Be aware of: Tiredness, Heart and Pulse Rate Change, Impatience and Anxiety, Belching and Rumbling of the Abdomen, Heavy Feeling or Upset Stomach, Discharge from Nose and Throat. And remember, the information in this guide is not a substitute for medical help.

21

How can we stay away from junk food?

Wouldn't it be a million dollar trick if we can do it? It will solve America's number one problem. The junk food is one of the major reasons for obesity and related diseases. Yes, it is possible. Here's how.

When you eat junk food; do *kapalbhati* just after eating the food to a count 10 or maximum 20? It really works. Be careful not to overdo it. You can end up with upset stomach.

However, it is not to suggest that you eat junk food and then do *kapalbhati*. But junk food is a reality of life and we are dealing with it rather than ignoring it. No doubt that eating healthy is the way to go. There is no substitute for healthy diet.

NOTE: Of course, another common sense way to handle junk food is eating healthy when hungry and junk food only when not hungry or full. Suppress appetite by enjoying healthy foods.

About the Author

Dr. Sukhraj S. Dhillon has an advanced degree in life sciences and molecular biology from the west and a fascination with yoga, breathing, religion and spirituality from the east crafted out of studies at Yale University, U.S.A. and Punjab University, India. Therefore, he is uniquely qualified to present Eastern and Western synthesis of health issues. He has published over 12 books and 40 research papers, and has expressed his views in the news media and workshops. He has been the President, Chairman of the board, and life-trustee of a non-profit religious organization and has expressed his views in the congregation and at international seminars. Most of his titles are now available at **Amazon Kindle**, **Barnes & Noble** and other book seller.